Understanding *Amae*:
The Japanese Concept of Need-love

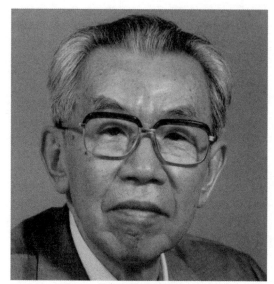

Takeo Doi, M.D.

The Collected Papers of
Twentieth-Century Japanese Writers
on Japan

VOLUME 1

Collected Papers

of

TAKEO DOI

Understanding *Amae*:
The Japanese Concept of Need-love

GLOBAL
ORIENTAL

Series: COLLECTED PAPERS OF TWENTIETH-CENTURY JAPANESE WRITERS ON JAPAN

Volume 1
Takeo Doi: Understanding *Amae*: The Japanese Concept of Need-love

First published in 2005 by
GLOBAL ORIENTAL LTD
PO Box 219
Folkestone
Kent CT20 2WP
UK

www.globaloriental.co.uk

ISBN 1-901903-28-1

British Library Cataloguing in Publication Data
a CIP catalogue entry for this book is available
From the British Library

Set in 11 on 12 point by Bookman, Hayes, Middlesex
Printed and bound in England by Antony Rowe Ltd., Chippenham, Wilts

Contents

Preface

It is a great honor to have had Professor S. Hirakawa write a very informative foreword to this Collection of my papers. We have known each other for many years and it was my good fortune indeed that I was once asked to participate in very exciting discussions of world literature at international conferences he organized. I should emphasize here that this Collection itself would not have come into being were it not for his strong encouragement and recommendation. I therefore want to avail myself of this occasion to express my heartfelt thanks for his friendship.

Most of the papers in this Collection were written for presentation at various international meetings during the past half century. The subjects dealt with here are as varied as the titles of each paper suggest. Interestingly, however, all the papers take up *amae* in one way or another as a central concept for discussion, thus throwing light in turn on the concept of *amae* from various angles. In fact this Collection will serve as a complement to my earlier book, *The Anatomy of Dependence* (Kodansha International, 1973), which made *amae* known to the English-speaking public for the first time. Again, speaking of *amae*, and as an additional reference, it may not be out of place to mention here my good friend Frank Johnson's scholarly work, *Dependency and Japanese Socialization, Psychoanalytic and Anthropological Investigations into Amae* (New York University Press, 1993) for further reference. Also, may I recommend another book of mine, *The Anatomy of Self* (Kodansha International, 1986), for further elucidation of the conceptual world where *amae* is viable?

I sincerely hope that even those who never heard of *amae* before will stumble on something here that can be said to be almost familiar, though it possibly was never acknowledged as such. Now, in closing, let me thank those colleagues and friends who either provided me with occasions to contribute papers or strongly encouraged me to do so. Some of them are dead now. May their souls rest in peace. Finally, I want to thank Ms Ayako Nakagawa who typed many of the papers presented here, even digging up some reference material and also did invaluable service in preparing the indexes.

TAKEO DOI
Tokyo
November 2004

PUBLISHER'S NOTE

Given the fact that over the last half century Professor Doi's writings have appeared mostly in American journals, it seemed most appropriate to republish them here in their original form, conforming with US spelling and punctuation norms. Elsewhere, British English conventions have been applied or respected.

Foreword

BY SUKEHIRO HIRAKAWA
Professor Emeritus, Tokyo University
Honorary Member, MLA

D r Takeo Doi with his *Amae no kōzō* (Tokyo, Kōbundō publishers, 1971) has had an immense impact both on the psychiatric world of specialists and on the Japanese readership in general. By 2003 the book had achieved a sale of almost one-and-a-half million copies.

Then, what is *amae*? Doi explains the meaning of the Japanese word as follows: *amae* is the noun form of '*amaeru*', an intransitive verb meaning 'to depend and presume upon another's benevolence' (Doi, 1956). This word has the same root as *amai*, an adjective that means 'sweet'. Thus, *amaeru* has a distinct feeling of sweetness and is generally used to describe a child's attitude or behaviour towards his parents, particularly his mother. Doi believes that there is no single word in English equivalent to *amaeru*, though this does not mean that the psychology of *amae* is totally alien to the people of English-speaking countries. I am sure that you will find among children in English-speaking countries those who *amaeru* – that is, his or hers is a dependent nature always seeking for someone on which to lean. However, as *amae* was first presented by Doi himself as a key concept for understanding the Japanese personality structure, it has sometimes been interpreted as something peculiarly Japanese. This interpretation is not correct.

Two years after the publication of the Japanese original, *Amae no kōzō* was translated into English. The English title given by the translator John Bester was *The Anatomy of Dependence* (Tokyo, Kodansha International, 1973). Ezra Vogel wrote in his review: '(*The Anatomy of Dependence* is) perhaps the first book by a Japanese trained in psychiatry to have an impact on Western psychiatric thinking.' Then followed the German, Korean, French, Italian, Chinese, Indonesian and Thai translations. The German translation was entitled *Amae: Freiheit in Geborgenheit* (1982) and the French translation *Le Jeu de l'Indulgence* (1988). The German and the French translators gave these different titles, probably trying to avoid the negative impression that the word *dependence* implies in the title of the English version. Quite a lot of confusion concerning the key concept has arisen, and clarification is necessary.

Fortunately, good ways are now open to those who wish to understand correctly what Doi means by the psychology of *amae*. Here in his *Collected*

Papers, all that Dr Doi has written in English is published for the first time in a single volume. For more than half a century Dr Doi has actively attended many international conferences where he explains in various ways his concept of *amae*. His are papers of ingenious skill, full of shrewd psychological insights. They have always been welcomed and have been published in academic journals throughout the world. Twenty-seven papers are brought together here, and are placed chronologically. Though not a psychiatrist myself, I very much appreciate Dr Doi's writings both in Japanese and English, and I feel privileged to be asked to write a Foreword for this volume.

Takeo Doi was born in 1920. He graduated from Tokyo University in 1942. After The Second World War, he went to study at the Meninger School of Psychiatry in Topeka, Kansas, in 1950, which was to mark the beginning of his frequent visits to the United States. While serving as psychiatrist-in-chief at St Luke's International Hospital, Tokyo, Doi initiated seminars in psychotherapy at Tokyo University School of Medicine. He then became professor at Tokyo University during the years of the students' rebellion. Later, he was appointed the director of the National Institute of Mental Health, Tokyo. His seven books concerning *amae* were published by the Kōbundō press between 1971 and 2001. His eight-volume selected writings, *Doi Takeo senshū*, were published by the Iwanami shoten in 2000.

Let me add some personal observations of mine which will explain partially the success of Doi's books among Japanese general readers. I am a comparative culture scholar, and am very much interested in the psychology of *amae*. The reasons are mainly as follows.

As I have said, *amae* is considered one of the key concepts which provide an understanding in depth of many aspects of Japanese culture. Doi himself once taught depth psychology using the novels of Natsume Sōseki at Waseda University. (See his *The Psychological World of Natsume Sōseki*, 1976.) He tried a literary analysis, applying the concept of *amae* to other works of literature as well. One of his successful applications in this direction is 'A Japanese Interpretation of Erich Segal's *Love Story*' (1972) which appears in this volume. On our initiative, together with Dr Doi as a commentator, a dozen scholars from Japan, Korea and European countries held international symposia to analyse works of literature, using the key concept of *amae*. The results of those conferences were published in *Amae de bungaku o toku* (*Analysis of Literature, using the concept of* amae, Hirakawa and Tsuruta ed., Tokyo, Shinyōsha, 1996). Psychological worlds of dependence of Kafka, Dostoevski, Yi Sang, Shiga Naoya and other Japanese writers have been elucidated to a surprising degree.

I am not sure if Dr Doi agrees with the following, but it seems to me that the world of Japanese *haiku* always takes for granted something unspoken in order to make sense of what is literally conveyed there. *Haiku* poets as well as *haiku* readers are accomplices of silence: brought up in a culturally homogeneous society, the Japanese share unspoken connotations to a greater degree. They therefore unconsciously presume upon another's sympathetic understanding. Is this not a kind of *amae* psychology? There is a part of non-verbal communication in the world of *haiku*. Both *haiku* poets and readers understand the greater hidden part of an iceberg, by catching sight of the visible part of it. Let me quote a *haiku* by Bashō:

Kiku no ka ya   Nara ni wa furuki   hotoke-tachi

At Nara;
The smell of chrysanthemums,
The ancient images of Buddha.

Nara is an ancient capital of Japan with many Buddhist temples. The ordinary connection is with the smell of incense. The poetical effect comes from the unexpected connection between the smell of chrysanthemums and the ancient Buddhas, which is so refreshing and life-resurrecting. Sharing readers' tacit understanding of traditional images of Nara, its old temples and venerable statues, the poet is able to open up a new vista by introducing a clear element of nature. Bashō expresses in a short space of seventeen syllables a fresh sensation of sight and odour peculiar to the Autumn.

I had better quote another example from a masterpiece of Western literature to prove the efficacy of this new analytical approach. Having translated the *Divine Comedy* into Japanese, I made an attempt to apply the concept of *amae* to the emotional relationship between the master-guide (Virgil) and his disciple-follower (Dante) in the *Divine Comedy*. The possibility of applying this key concept to the particular situation presupposes a certain resemblance in the mother-child relationship, both in Italy and in Japan. (The situation is different in countries with mainly Protestant traditions, the cult of a mother force being practically absent because of the reformed Christianity.) When a sound emotional relationship is established between mother and child, it is easy to develop a constructive relationship between teacher and pupil.

Taking it for granted that a teacher appears to a young child as a substitute for his or her mother, and that the teacher-pupil relationship is somewhat similar to the mother-child relationship (both being rich in *amae*), I tried to analyse the verbal and non-verbal communications between Virgil and Dante during their journey through Hell and through Purgatory. The psychological analysis of the relationship between the teacher Virgil and the pupil Dante in the fictional world of the *Divine Comedy*, so strikingly similar to the mother-child connection, shows clearly the tendency to search for indulgent love (*amae*) on the part of the author Dante. In his masterpiece Dante as a *dramatis persona* seeks to be babied! Among Japanese female readers the most popular figure in Dante's poem is Virgil, and the fascination for Virgil (not the real Latin poet Vergilius of *Aeneid* but Virgilio of the *Divina Commedia*) is explained satisfactorily when the anatomy of dependence of Dante is analysed through Doi's theory.[*] Dante as a *dramatis persona* depends so much on Virgil.

In fact, I have enjoyed Dr Doi's interdisciplinary friendship for over a quarter of a century. His comments have opened new vistas many times. When I heard his remarks on the meaning of non-verbal communication between Virgil and Dante, I had an intimation like that of Freudian psychoanalysis that had once revolutionized literary studies. I am sure that Doi's *amae* theory would have wider repercussions outside Dr Doi's specialized field of psychiatry, if applied to other disciplines as well. Is not Japan's love-hate relationship with the West worth a much closer attention from this psychological point of view?

I am very glad that the English papers of Doi *sensei*, to whom I owe so much, should be brought into a wider stream of intelligent reading.

* S. Hirakawa, 'Anatomia della dipendenza di Dante: Un'interpretazione giapponese dei rapporti affettivi fra maestro e discepolo nella *Divina Commedia*' was published in *Giappone, Sensi e Sentimenti*, atti del xvii convegno di studi, (AISTUGIA), M.C.S. Edizioni, Firenze, 1994.

First published in *American Journal of Psychiatry,* Vol.111, No.9, pp.691-695, 1955

① Some Aspects of Japanese Psychiatry*

I t is a great honor to be invited to your convention to deliver a speech on Japanese psychiatry. When Major Yessler told me about this invitation early in April, I was hesitant to accept it, because I knew I was not well qualified to say anything definite about Japanese psychiatry. I came only recently to psychiatry, that is, in 1950, after seven years' experience in medicine including three years' service in the Japanese Army. And since I was in the United States for psychiatric training from 1950 to 1952, I have actually been with Japanese psychiatry for less than two years. One can hardly say that this length of time is adequate to make a survey of as vast a field as Japanese psychiatry. Therefore, I consulted two professors of psychiatry, Dr. Muramatsu of Nagoya University and Dr. Suwa of Hokkaido University, to see if they would deliver a speech instead. They have both been trained in the United States and are far better qualified for this task because of their long and distinguished service in Japanese psychiatry. Both of them, however, said that they could not possibly come to Tokyo at this time, and I had to decide to come to the task alone. I want you therefore to know from the beginning that what I am going to tell you is necessarily limited and can hardly cover even those things of importance in Japanese psychiatry.

I think it will be proper to begin a talk on Japanese psychiatry by some reflection on its history. It is known that Dr. Baelz, a German internist invited by the Japanese government to help establish Tokyo University Medical School, lectured on modern psychiatry for the first time in Japan in 1879. But the regular course in the medical curriculum was initiated in 1886 by Dr. Sakaki, the first Japanese professor of psychiatry. Succeeding Dr. Sakaki as professor of psychiatry was Dr. Kure, who returned to Japan in 1901 after four years' study in Germany under Kraepelin and Nissl, and it was he, we may say, who determined the course of Japanese psychiatry for the following fifty years up to this date. Dr. Kure found that neuropathology in particular, which he learned from Nissl, attracted a number of bright students, who in turn pursued this discipline with such intensity and enthusiasm that it has become the most active field in Japanese psychiatry. But I do not want you to have the impression that

* Presented May 4, 1954, at the Neuropsychiatric Conference, FEC, U.S. Army Hospital, 8167th Army Unit, Tokyo.

Japanese psychiatry has been solely under the influence of the German school, for there have been a few professors of psychiatry who have studied in France or the United States, though they have exerted comparatively little influence. Among them I mention only Dr. Marui who was professor of psychiatry at Tohoku University. He for the first time introduced psychoanalytical theories to Japanese psychiatry some thirty years ago after his study in the United States under Adolf Meyer and later established a branch of the International Society of Psychoanalysis in Japan, but the over-all result of his pioneer work was anything but a success. I shall return to this topic later. In this connection, Dr. Morita, who was professor of psychiatry at Jikei University, should also be mentioned. He was the first Japanese psychiatrist who became intensely interested in psychotherapy and devised a special method of psychotherapy which starts with confinement to bed in isolation and goes on to occupational therapy along with supportive explanation and counseling. This brand of psychotherapy was said to be effective for a type of neurosis called *shinkeishitsu* and was followed at various university clinics, notably Kyushu University. (*Shinkeishitsu* literally means nervousness, but denotes hypochondriac personality rather than just nervousness.) As a matter of fact, Dr. Morita's method is still in use at many places, and was reported by Drs. Jacobson and Berenber at the 1952 meeting of The American Psychiatric Association.[1] Now the interesting thing is that Dr. Marui, interpreter of psychoanalysis to Japanese psychiatry, and Dr. Morita, founder of the new school of psychotherapy, were engaged in very hot arguments at the conventions in 1930, '31, and '32, on the relative therapeutic value of psychoanalysis and Morita therapy. It is remembered that this verbal duel between two professors was most exciting to all who attended the conventions, but no one ever really knew which side won the battle.

I mentioned above that American psychiatry had little influence on Japanese psychiatry, but this has not been true since the end of The Second World War. Japanese psychiatrists, hungry for new knowledge, have attempted to test and absorb whatever they found good in American psychiatry. But they have left one thing undigested so far: that is dynamic orientation which is so essential, as I see it, to American psychiatry. (Some of you may object to the adjective 'essential', but will not deny that dynamic orientation is the most prominent feature of present American psychiatry.) To give you a general idea of the impact which dynamic orientation has had on the minds of Japanese psychiatrists, I think I shall do best by quoting from the keynote address by Dr. Uchimura entitled 'The Past and Future of Japanese Psychiatry', which was given at the 50th convention of the Japanese Neuropsychiatric Association in 1953. But before quoting from his speech, let me say a few words about Dr. Uchimura himself so that you may understand better the weight his speech had on Japanese psychiatrists. Dr. Uchimura has been professor of psychiatry at Tokyo University for the past 18 years and has been the most prominent figure in Japanese psychiatry. He was trained at the Institute for Psychiatric Research in Munich, Germany, from 1925 to 1927 under the eminent Dr. Spielmeyer. (It may interest you to know that Dr. Lawrence S. Kubie, now practicing psychoanalysis in New York was in the same institute at the time when Dr. Uchimura was there and they became very good friends.) Dr. Uchimura's scientific interest then was naturally drawn to neuropathology, like other leading Japanese psychiatrists, and he has contributed numerous important papers to that field, ranging from mid-brain pathology, pathogenesis of epilepsy to cerebral pathology caused by the atomic bomb. But his interest was not limited to neuropathology alone, rather he has kept a keen interest in every field of psychiatry, having published various papers on themes such as the Ainu race and its Imu, incidence of psychosis among the Japanese population, as well as conducting many research groups in twin study, electroencephalography, and psychosurgery. It should also be noted here that he is a great teacher and has educated more psychiatrists than any other professor. As a matter of fact, twelve contemporary professors of psychiatry are his former pupils. (I may add that the one who is reading this paper is also one of his many pupils.)

Now returning to his keynote address at the 50th convention in 1953, Dr. Uchimura's statement about American psychiatry is as follows:

> I was really surprised to know that American psychiatry had taken in so much from psychoanalytical theories and had also put a great emphasis on clinical psychological testing. . . . I think it is a great task for Japanese psychiatrists to understand correctly what dynamic psychiatry is and to face it with a critical mind. . . . Among several doubts that I have about dynamic psychiatry, the greatest one concerns its overestimation of childhood experiences and milieu, especially its attempt to explain adult behavior or symptoms in terms of those experiences, which I find far-fetched and lacking in substantial validation.

In spite of this criticism, however, he does not oppose the practice of psychotherapy, based on dynamic principles if it is the thing which really helps the patient, but here again he ponders about whether or not any unbiased scientific study has ever been done to test dynamics or psychoanalytical psychotherapy against another brand of psychotherapy, so that we may recognize the unique significance of dynamic psychother-apy. Now you may wonder what sort of psychopathology Japanese psychiatrists generally entertain, if most of them reject analytical psychopathology as fictitious. One group takes to German psychopathol-ogy represented by Karl Jaspers, now a famous philosopher, and another group takes to French psychopathology descending from Pierre Janet. The former finds its followers mostly among Tokyo University psychiatrists and the latter mostly among Kyoto University psychiatrists.

Having oriented you to the prevailing academic atmosphere in Japanese psychiatry, I will proceed to a brief description of the present status of

Japanese mental hygiene. By this I mean the condition of mental hospitals as well as the system for training psychiatrists and adjunctive staff. The estimated nation-wide population of the mentally ill in Japan, which excludes neurotics, but includes severe character disorder, is about 3,500,000, and one-fifth, 700,000 consists of psychotics. Among these psychotics some 150,000 are believed to need hospitalization, while the total number of beds available for these patients amounts only to 27,000, i.e., only 18% of the beds needed, and this figure, by the way, constitutes 7.19% of all hospital beds in Japan. Further, if you compare the ratio of mental hospital beds to the total population of various countries in the world, that of Japan ranks with the lowest, namely, 2.2 per 10,000, whereas that of the United States is 50, which is the top figure. I do not believe that this incredible shortage of mental hospital beds can be explained simply on the basis of the low economic status of Japan. I personally feel that the incentive of the public to promote mental hygiene has never been great here and the psychiatrists also on their part have not been so enthusiastic about enlightening the public as they are about academic research. It should be pointed out that the Japanese psychiatrists as a whole are very research-minded, but not so profession-conscious as their American colleagues are. This is reflected, I think, in their failure to establish the formal residency program and the specialty board, the purpose of which is solely to maintain the high level of the profession. For instance, almost all young physicians who, after internship, take psychiatric training at the university clinics, do start or prepare themselves for some research within a year or so. Likewise, the fact that the Japanese psychiatrists show a considerable interest in psychometrics points in the same direction. This being the case, it seems to me that in Japan clinical psychologists will never enjoy an independent position as they do in the United States. This is entirely an opposite picture to that of the United States, where clinical psychologists not infrequently turn to a profession of psychotherapy, apart from their chief concern in psychometrics and its related research. Speaking about the training of psychiatrists, it should also be mentioned that making two different professions of psychiatry and neurology has not been the practice here, but there recently seems to be a steady movement in that direction, particularly on the part of internists who have specialized in neurology. Incidentally, the total number of Japanese psychiatrists is estimated to be about 800, a very small number, although there is a tendency to rapid increase in recent years. Now as for the training of adjunctive staff such as psychiatric nurses, attendants, occupational therapists, there are no systematic courses or training centers for them at present.

I want to add here, in passing, a few words about the present status of child psychiatry in Japan. There are now a few research centers for child psychiatry, but at the time of writing no medical school has a professor of child psychiatry on its staff. The child guidance clinic was introduced into postwar Japan according to the pattern in the United States and there are now about 110 clinics scattered throughout Japan, staffed mostly with clinical psychologists and social workers and only in rare instances with psychiatrists. At the present time these clinics chiefly serve as the temporary placement centers for orphans as well as mentally retarded children, and there is very little practice of guidance. This can be attributed to the fact that very few members have had enough training for the professional skill of guidance or counseling. As a matter of fact, psychotherapy in general, has not yet established itself as a profession in Japan, its practice being mainly limited to moral support which the physician gives the patient casually, unless it takes a particular form like Morita therapy.

Now I will turn to the discussion of Japanese psychoanalysis. About this subject a very interesting and informative article by Dr. James Clark Moloney, entitled, 'Understanding the Paradox of Japanese Psycho-analysis', appeared in a recent issue of the *International Journal of Psychoanalysis*. In this article the author contends, judging from various articles which appeared in the *Tokyo Journal of Psychoanalysis*, that the practice of psychoanalysts in Japan is quite different from what it is in the Occidental countries, being contaminated, so to speak, by the Japanese way of life which all Japanese analysts share. This remark is interesting when you compare it with Drs. Jacobson and Berenberg's interpretation of Morita therapy as an embodiment of the Japanese way of life. I will quote Dr. Moloney's conclusions:

> . . . it is evident that these [Japanese] scientists entertain precisely the same attitude towards the individual as is expressed in *Kokutai No Hongi* [the name of the textbook meaning the cardinal principles of the national entity of Japan]. Without question they subscribe to the concept of coevality with heaven, earth, and emperor, and they regard the individual as a segment of the national entity of Japan. . . . In the adaptation accomplished by the Japanese psychoanalysts, the conscious ego becomes synonymous with an awareness of the cardinal principles of the national entity of Japan.

Speaking of the national entity of Japan in terms of coevality with heaven, earth, and emperor is quite out of date in postwar democratized Japan and nobody now believes in it [I hope so] but nevertheless Dr. Moloney's observations are, in my opinion, essentially correct and still apply as far as the basic mentality of the Japanese people is concerned. However, if he draws the conclusion from these observations that Japanese psychoanalysts necessarily and simply because of their being Japanese cannot grasp the true meaning of psychoanalysis, I cannot agree with him. To state this in simple words, what is really wrong with these Japanese psychoanalysts is their lack of proper psychoanalytic training. As a matter of fact, Dr. Kosawa, a former disciple of Dr. Marui who is the founder of the Japanese Psychoanalytical Society, is the only one who has had any form of training, and he has had only three months of training analysis while he was in Austria in 1932, which can hardly be said to be adequate according to the standard that the International Society of Psychoanalysis sets up. I have been in close contact with him for the past few years and know how well read he is in psychoanalytical literature and theories, but I should say that he is seriously handicapped in treating patients. Incidentally, he is a devout Buddhist and there seems to be no distinction in his mind between his religion and psychoanalysis. Hence, you may suspect that his approach to patients must be quite authoritarian, which it is; however, it may be said that his attitude is matriarchal rather than patriarchal according to his religious or psychoanalytical convictions. Now supposing that my theory that what is wrong with the Japanese psychoanalysts is their deficient training is right, the question remains as to what would become of the Japanese psychiatrists or lay people when they undergo the proper course of training analysis. Would they be more Occidental after analysis than before, as may be derived from Dr. Moloney's tacit assumption that the goal of psychoanalysis is coexistent or identical with that of Occidental individualism? To phrase the question in another way, would those Occidentals, American or European, who undergo analysis become more Occidental or individualistic by analysis? This question is as interesting and thought-provocative as it sounds a little funny, but since it involves the relationship of psychoanalysis as a science to psychoanalysis as a potential *Weltanschauung* or ideology and is not subject to a simple answer, I will not discuss it further.

In discussing Japanese psychoanalysis above I came across the problem of cultural differences between the Occident and the Orient. I think this problem, especially its bearing upon different types of mental patients, has lately drawn considerable attention front American psychiatrists and cultural anthropologists and you may therefore be interested in hearing the Japanese psychiatrist's opinions on this matter. I regret to say, however, that I have no definite opinion except a few unorganized thoughts, nor have I conducted any relevant research myself. As I understand it, the psychiatric team of Nagoya University is doing some research along this line with the help of Dr. DeVos, an American clinical psychologist, and another American cultural anthropologist is expected to join the team this coming autumn. So far we have not seen any published report from them on this particular problem, and we look forward to seeing it soon. But I have an apprehension that if their research relies solely on psychometrics, and formal interpretations by the standard which is nothing else but a deduction from a large number of answers given by Occidental people, they miss a subtle, peculiarly Japanese trait which they are looking for, since they set out with a working hypothesis that there may be such a Japanese trait. Of course I do not mean that there is no possibility of getting a typically Japanese reaction on psychological testing, but I am afraid that what is most typically Japanese, if there is such a quality, will be lost through psychometrics as it is constructed now. The reason for my apprehension is very simple, that the typical psychology of a given nation can be learned only through familiarity with its native language. The language comprises everything which is intrinsic to the soul of a nation and therefore stands for the best projective test there is for each nation. It is too obvious to say that psychiatrists in Occidental countries do not solely rely on psychometrics for psychological examination of their patients even if psychometrics turns out to be quite sensitive. How then could it be fit for determining a subtle national trait of a foreign country? I may add that a sociological study of a foreign nation also cannot have any depth without the knowledge of the language. For instance when you say with Dr. Moloney that the Japanese 'regard the individual as a segment of the national entity of Japan', how can you differentiate it from other totalitarian concepts such as exemplified in Nazism or Communism? Or is there no difference at all between them, so far as they are totalitarian? I am the one who takes the view that there is a difference psychologically and sociologically in the degree and quality of being totalitarian, subtle and elusive as it may be. At any rate I would strongly recommend to you, if you are interested in getting to the bottom of Japanese psychology, that you thoroughly familiarize yourself with the Japanese language and associate with as many non-English-speaking Japanese people as possible. This must be a *sine qua non* for a complete study of the Japanese culture.

I have tried to give you the origin and the prevailing academic atmosphere in Japanese psychiatry, a description of the slow development of mental hygiene and the unsuccessful movement of Japanese psychoanalysis, and have drawn your attention to the problem and difficulty of studying the Japanese culture and its bearing upon psychiatry. I have deliberately avoided discussing in detail numerous contributions by the Japanese psychiatrists, most of which are in the organic field, mainly because I am not as familiar with them as I should be.

Now in closing, I want to express again my deep appreciation for this invitation, which I consider not only as a great personal honor, but an honor to the entire body of Japanese psychiatry, since this is the first time, to my knowledge, that a Japanese psychiatrist has been invited to address a convention of American psychiatrists.

NOTES

1.   *Am. J. Psychiat.*, Nov. 1952.

First published in *Western Speed*, Berkley, Spring 1956

② Japanese Language as an Expression of Japanese Psychology

To begin with, let me say that I am a Japanese, born and educated in Japan. Though I am going to talk about the Japanese language, I am not a student of the Japanese language or of a related field. I am a psychiatrist and have come to this country for psychoanalytic training.

My interest in certain aspects of the Japanese language arose as a result of my two years' training in psychiatry in this country (1950-52), and my return to Japan, where I practiced psychiatry for three years. Because of this background, I have become acutely aware of a question which interests many other persons – the question whether or not the psychopathology of Japanese patients differs noticeably from that of American patients. Almost every psychiatrist assumes a difference because of the different cultural backgrounds. But articulating the difference is not an easy job. One day it struck me that any differences between the psychopathologies of the two different nationalities must exist in an embryonic form in the different characteristics of the two languages. This conception derived from the following considerations: first, any difference between the psychopathologies of two nationalities must be a reflection of some difference in the national characteristics; and second, the characteristics of a given nation must be intrinsic in its language. Although, so far as I know, no author has followed this line of reasoning, despite the many books and articles that have been published on the subject of Japanese psychology in this country, I felt, it was a valid approach. Later, when I took up Edward Sapir's book, *Language*,[1] and read the chapter, 'Language, Race, and Culture', I had to reconsider my ideas, because Sapir contends that it is impossible to prove a connection between language and national temperament. As a layman in the science of language, I could not evaluate or criticize his opinion and yet I felt suspicious about so categorical a viewpoint. It seemed to run contrary to the basic assumption under which psychiatrists work. We assume in interviewing a patient that the words and manner of his speech, intended to convey information, also express his mental status to the experienced observer. That is, in a given individual, we assume a connection between his language and his temperament. Why, then, can we not increase our understanding of the psychology of a whole people through an analysis of their language?

In considering more fully this idea, I found two writers who at least seemed not to contradict my theory – Ernst Cassirer and David Rapaport. I shall quote from both. Cassirer states, '(the names) are not designed to refer to substantiate things, independent entities which exist by themselves. They are determined by *human interests* and *human purposes* (italics mine). . . . For in the act of denomination we select, out of the multiplicity and diffusion of our sense data, certain fixed centers of perception.'[2] He cites as an example the following: 'The Greek and Latin terms for the moon, although they refer to the same object, do not express the same intention or concept. The Greek term (men) denotes the function of the moon to "measure" time: the Latin term (luna, luc-na) denotes the moon's lucidity or brightness.'

This opinion Rapaport seems to support from the psychoanalytic point of view. He states: 'The memorial connections, the conceptual belonging-ness, and the anticipations which have once arisen in the interplay of motivations and in the quest for the object which satisfies simultaneously several effective motives (over-determination), are not lost with the progress of psychological development; rather, by again and again recurring in approximately similar situations, they become structuralized and available as fixed tools, quasi-stationary apparatuses, for use in the thought process.'[3] Although Rapaport is not here talking specifically about language, yet a fixed tool 'for use in the thought process' is a function of language, and there is no reason not to apply it as a theoretical postulate to account for possible psychological meanings in the development and usage of different languages. Thus, to state my hypothesis succinctly in the light of these two authors, the characteristics of a given language may reflect some particular aspects of the interaction between early instinctual drives and the environment.

Now I turn to my analysis of some Japanese words, but I want to stress again that the analysis came first; only later did I wish to formulate a theoretical framework for my findings.

In the first place I would like to explain four Japanese intransitive verbs which are commonly used to express feelings and represent emotive behavior. I emphasize that they are intransitive verbs, not descriptive adjectives. They express subjective feelings and actions when used. The first, *amaeru*, can be translated as 'to depend and presume upon another's love'. This word has the same root as *amai*, an adjective which corresponds to 'sweet'. Thus *amaeru* has a distinct feeling of sweetness, and is generally used to express a child's attitude toward an adult, especially his parents. I can think of no English word equivalent to *amaeru* except for 'spoil', which, however, is a transitive verb and definitely has a bad connotation; whereas the Japanese *amaeru* does not necessarily have a bad connotation, although we say we should not let a youngster *amaeru* too much. I think most Japanese adults have a dear memory of the taste of sweet dependency as a child and, consciously or unconsciously, carry a life-long nostalgia for it.

9

Two other words closely related to *amaeru* are *suneru* and *higamu*. These are also intransitive verbs, again used chiefly regarding a child's behavior, and they are counterparts to the sweetness of *amaeru*. When a child does *suneru*, he pouts and sulks because he feels his parents do not let him *amaeru* enough. Externally he can become demanding to the extent of a temper tantrum, but the essence of *suneru* is not an open demanding; rather, a subtle soliciting of another's love, which he wants to possess by himself alone. You may say there is a hint of jealousy here, but the reflection of sibling rivalry is more apparent in our next word, *higamu*. When a child does *higamu*, he feels himself unfairly treated in comparison to others and very often suspects or anticipates that he is or will be rejected, even though it may not be the case – the budding of a paranoid feeling. We can and do use these words at times regarding an adult, but we necessarily imply that the man is childish.

There is one more Japanese intransitive verb, *kodawaru*, the English equivalent of which I cannot find. This is a very common word that we Japanese all know but when we try to explain its meaning we are surprised at the difficulty. Indeed, I have come across a few foreign residents in Japan who have lived there many years and have never used or even heard of the word *kodawaru*, despite their excellent command of the Japanese language. Because *kodawaru* means a very subtle disturbance that takes place inside the minds of the Japanese people, they will never express it in the presence of strangers. The English translation would be something like 'to be subject to the notion of', and 'to be scrupulous about' or 'to be sensitive about' is perhaps the nearest English idiomatic expression. But *kodawaru* does not necessarily apply to a moral problem like scrupulosity; it is rather like a general obsession, though usually ego-syntonic and not ego-alien, and therefore more or less a preoccupation at the moment of its presence. The objects about which one does *kodawaru* can be varied, from simple innocent things, daily rituals, to physical sensations, suppressed grudges, or embarrassments toward somebody. It is easy to see that there can be all grades from benign *kodawaru*, so to speak, to severe obsession or hypochondriasis. Now the important thing about *kodawaru* is that it does not appear on the surface and those who have it rarely talk about it. Furthermore, even if one senses another's *kodawari* (the noun of *kodawaru*), he usually does not try to remove it, again because of his own *kodawari*. Here, you see, the essence of well-known Japanese politeness, which serves the purpose of protecting privacy.

Next I want to explain the negative form of the intransitive verb *sumu*, that is, *sumanai*. The meaning of *sumu* is to end, to be finished or to be settled, but its negative form has various usages besides its literal meaning. This expression can also be used on those occasions when you say in English, 'I feel guilty', 'I am sorry', 'Thank you'. You hear this expression often, indeed, in Japan. Of course I do not mean that *sumanai* can be equated with the three English expressions, but the word can indicate a peculiarly Japanese reaction to the three instances when three different English expressions are used. First, 'I feel guilty' conveys the meaning that you have offended something or somebody and for this you are troubled in your conscience. But the Japanese feels a little differently in such a situation. He feels that he has not done as he was supposed to do, therefore something remains unended; hence, the expression *sumanai*. In other words, *sumanai* conveys the sense of failure with an air of apology rather than that of guilt.

This explains why the same *sumanai* is used in cases where the English expression 'I am sorry' is adequate. But here again there is a difference between the two, because 'I am sorry' always has a connotation of sympathy or pity, whereas *sumanai* never has this feeling. To express this sympathetic aspect of 'I am sorry', there is another Japanese phrase, which we use only when we are sure that we have no part whatsoever in the cause of another's grief. I think the most puzzling is the last application of *sumanai*, when you simply say 'thank you'. This will be best understood if you consider the occasions when you say, besides a simple 'thank you', something like, 'You shouldn't have done this', 'I am sorry to put you to so much trouble', etc. *Sumanai* used on such occasions goes one step farther than these English expressions, and conveys again the feeling of failure in the sense that 'I shouldn't have let you do this', instead of 'you shouldn't have done this'. It is noteworthy how often and almost invariably we Japanese use *sumanai* in cases where we want to thank others.

It is then an entirely legitimate question to ask why the Japanese fuss so much about the sense of failure when one should be perfectly delighted with the kindness rendered to him. This is because kindness in Japanese society tends to be obligating more often than not. It means that 'since I failed to prevent you from doing this, I am indebted to you'. To avoid misunderstanding, let me emphasize that an act of kindness in Japan is not meant to obligate people; it is something very natural and spontaneous, perhaps more spontaneous than it can be in American society. Despite or perhaps because of its spontaneity, neither does Japanese kindness bear the quality of being 'free'. I mean by 'free' the state of being gratis. I think this fact – that kindness or giving is not entirely free or gratis in Japanese society – is somewhat related to our lack of the concept of freedom in the Occidental sense, though we do have the concepts of self-indulgence or self-choice. Of course the Occidental usage of the word 'freedom' very often includes these, too, but there seems to be something more to it, especially when you say that one is a free, independent person. And I strongly feel that this concept of freedom was born from the fact that here kindness or giving can be free or gratis; that is, no obligation is incurred, no strings are attached, so that one doesn't have to feel *sumanai*. I do not mean that kindness or giving in American society is always free and gratis or that you never experience *sumanai*. On the contrary, you do so often, in my observation, although this is experienced and expressed as a feeling of

11

guilt. Incidentally this is what I miss in Ruth Benedict's excellent analysis of this feeling of indebtedness in the Japanese mind, which we call *on* in Japanese, because she somehow gives an impression that this is a particularly Japanese phenomenon, something that you can never expect here.[4] Nor do I propose here that the present usage of 'guilt' is the exact equivalent of our *sumanai*, although a detailed discussion of the concept of guilt is beyond the purpose of my paper. I only suggest that the concept of Japanese *sumanai* may throw light on the Occidental concepts of 'guilt' or 'freedom'.

I should like now to explain the common root which appears in a large number of Japanese adjectives and verbs regarding human feelings, character, or behavior. For instance, take such adjectives as guilty, capricious, fond, queer, crazy, irritable, narrow-minded, tender-minded, short-tempered, depressed, apprehensive, inclined, reluctant, genial, impatient, oppressive, sensible, generous, frank, smart, etc. Most of the Japanese words that correspond to these English words have the same root, *ki*. The word *ki* came originally from the Chinese language and in various contexts has many meanings, such as breath, air, weather, vapor, vigor, temperament. In this respect it corresponds to 'spirit' and may illustrate an interesting parallel between Oriental and Occidental usages of the concept.

What I want to point out here, however, is the way in which the Japanese people compounded many adjectives about human nature on this simple common root *ki*, so much so that they evolve a new concept out of *ki*, apart from its original meanings in Chinese. The interesting thing is that in these adjectives *ki* is grammatically treated as the subject; very often the real subject or person to whom the particular adjective is referred is not mentioned. For instance, instead of 'I feel depressed' we can say 'the *ki* sinks or rottens'. Likewise we prefer the expression 'you get in the *ki*' to 'I am fond of you' or 'I am pleased with you'. Again the common expression for 'I feel guilty' would be 'the *ki* reproaches or is not satisfied'. Instead of saying that he is crazy or insane, we more often say that his *ki* is queer or out of order. I could cite many more examples.

Let us consider what is implied in this impersonal way of expressing emotions and feelings. For myself, I cannot but feel that there is an indication of peculiar emotional autonomy as well as isolation, inasmuch as *ki* is always treated as the subject. It may imply that we are resigned to the fact that we always yield to our emotions and find ourselves quite often at their mercy. I have tacitly equated *ki* with emotion, and that is not too far from the truth. But there is a difference: *ki* as the common root plays various roles in various word-combinations, whereas 'emotion' remains a generic term. Indeed, there is an apparent contradiction in the usage of *ki* from case to case. To cite the most obvious example, the *ki* of guilt that refuses to be satisfied and the *ki* in self-indulgence where one behaves according to his *ki* stand conceptually opposite. Yet this is so only if you take *ki* as a generic term to represent a structure or system in the mind; for *ki* in Japanese usage does not represent emotion as isolated from reason or conscience, or vice versa, nor does it correspond to any of the three psychic structures, ego, super-ego and id, as conceptualized in psychoanalytic thinking. Rather, *ki* is the mind in action; it indicates the intentional or tendential essence of mind, whatever role it may play at the moment. A Japanese saying illustrates this point very well. Suppose one does another just a small favor which does not mean much materially, or that one repays a debt so small that both persons can easily forget about it; then the one says to the other, '*ki* is mind'. He means by this that his intention, rather than his action, is what really matters.

To me this concept of *ki* is extremely interesting in view of the fact that contemporary psychological thinking lays so much emphasis upon trying to arrive at a unitary theory of personality. Actually the original Japanese language – that is, before the Western impact on Japanese culture – did not have words to denote philosophical concepts like reason, conscience, will, or affect, and thus had a fairly unitary concept of personality as based on the concept of *ki*. But I must admit that this Japanese version of a unitary theory of personality without accompanying abstract concepts like reason, will, or affect is not entirely satisfactory, and I am sure that Occidental psychologists will not disagree.

These have been interpretations of some Japanese words that are very often used to express feelings and motions. I have analyzed each word and have not dealt with the psychological implications of the sentence structure in the Japanese language. Again I should like to emphasize that these words are common words, not technical terms, and describe common, not peculiar, behavior. Thus they may indicate something of the psychology common to the Japanese people.

NOTES

Dr. Doi, University of Tokyo, is a Fellow of the China Medical Board. This paper was read at the Center for Advanced Study in the Behavioral Sciences at Stanford University, and is based on an earlier paper delivered at the First Western Divisional Meeting of the American Psychiatric Association Joint meeting with the West Coast Psychoanalytic Societies, in San Francisco, October, 1955.
1.   Edward Sapir, *Language*, p. 217. A Harvest Book. New York: Harcourt. Brace & Co., 1949
2.   Ernst Cassirer, *An Essay on Man*, p. 173. New York: Doubleday Anchor Books, 1954.
3.   David Rapaport, 'The Conceptual Model of Psychoanalysts'. p. 241, In: *Psychoanalytic Psychiatry and Psychology* (ed. Robert P. Knight and Cyrus R. Friedman), New York, International Universities Press, Inc., 1954.
4.   Ruth Benedict, *The Chrysanthemum and the Sword*, Boston: Houghton Mifflin Co., 1946.

First published in Robert J. Smith and Richard K. Beardsley, eds, *Japanese Culture: Its Development and Characteristics*. Chicago Aldine Publishing Co., 1962. © Wenner-Gren Foundation for Anthropological Research, Inc.

③ *Amae*: A Key Concept for Understanding Japanese Personality Structure

I am particularly interested in the problem of personality and culture in modern Japan for two reasons. First, even though I was born and raised in Japan and had my basic medical training there, I have had further training in psychiatry and psychoanalysis in the United States, thus exposing myself for some time to a different culture from that of Japan. Second, I have had many opportunities of treating both Japanese and non-Japanese (mostly American) patients with psychotherapy. These experiences have led me to inquire into differences between Japanese and non-Japanese patients and also into the question of what is basic in Japanese character structure. In this paper I shall describe what I have found to be most characteristic in Japanese patients and then discuss its meaning in the context of Japanese culture.

The essence of what I am going to talk about is contained in one common Japanese word, '*amae*'. Let me therefore, first of all, explain the meaning of this word. *Amae* is the noun form of '*amaeru*', an intransitive verb that means 'to depend and presume upon another's benevolence' (Doi, 1956). This word has the same root as *amai*, an adjective that means 'sweet'. Thus *amaeru* has a distinct feeling of sweetness and is generally used to describe a child's attitude or behavior toward his parents, particularly his mother. But it can also be used to describe the relationship between two adults, such as the relationship between a husband and a wife or a master and a subordinate. I believe that there is no single word in English equivalent to *amaeru*, though this does not mean that the psychology of *amae* is totally alien to the people of English-speaking countries. I shall come back to this problem after describing some of the clinical material through which I came to recognize the importance of what this word *amae* signifies.

It was in my attempt to understand what goes on between the therapist and patient that I first came across the all-powerful drive of the patient's *amae*. There is a diagnostic term in Japanese psychiatry *shinkeishitsu*, which includes neurasthenia, anxiety neurosis, and obsessive neurosis. Morita, who first used *shinkeishitsu* as a diagnostic term, thought that these three types of neuroses had a basic symptom in common, *toraware*, which means 'to be bound or caught', as by some intense preoccupation. He considered *toraware* to be closely related to hypochondriacal fear and thought that this fear sets in motion a reciprocal intensification of attention and sensation. In psychoanalytic work with neurotic patients of the *shinkeishitsu* type I have also found *toraware* to be a basic symptom, but I have evolved a different formulation of its significance (see Doi, 1958). I have observed that during the course of psychotherapy the patient's *toraware* can easily turn into hypersensitivity in his relationship with the therapist. This hypersensitivity is best described by the Japanese word *kodawari*. *Kodawari* is the noun form of *kodawaru*, an intransitive verb meaning 'to be sensitive to minor things', 'to be inwardly disturbed over one's personal relationships'. In the state of *kodawari* one feels that he is not accepted by others, which suggests that *kodawari* results from the unsatisfied desire to *amaeru*. Thus *toraware* can be traced back through *kodawari* to *amae*. In my observations the patient's *toraware* usually receded when he became aware of his *amae* toward the therapist, which he had been warding off consciously and unconsciously up to then.

At first I felt that if the patient became fully aware of his *amae*, he would thereupon be able to get rid of his neurosis. But I was wrong in this assumption and came to observe another set of clinical phenomena following the patient's recognition of his *amae* (see Doi, 1960). Many patients confessed that they were then awakened to the fact that they had not 'possessed their self', had not previously appreciated the importance of their existence, and had been really nothing apart from their all-important desire to *amaeru*. I took this as a step toward the emergence of a new consciousness of self, inasmuch as the patient could then at least realize his previous state of 'no self'.

There is another observation that I should like to mention here. It is about the nature of guilt feelings of Japanese patients (see Doi, 1961). The word *sumanai* is generally used to express guilt feelings, and this word is the negative form of *sumu*, which means 'to end'. *Sumanai* literally means that one has not done as he was supposed to do, thereby causing the other person trouble or harm. Thus, it expresses more a sense of unfulfilled obligation than a confession of guilt, though it is generally taken as an indication that one feels guilty. When neurotic patients say *sumanai*, I have observed that there lies, behind their use of the word, much hidden aggression engendered by frustration of their wish to *amaeru*. So it seems that in saying *sumanai* they are in fact expressing their hidden concern lest they fall from the grace of *amae* because of their aggression. I think that this analysis of *sumanai* would also apply in essence to the use of this word by the ordinary Japanese in everyday life, but in the case of the neurotic patient *sumanai* is said with greater ambivalence. In other words, more than showing his feeling of being obligated, he tends to create a sense of obligation in the person to whom he makes his apology, thus 'forcing' that person eventually to cater to his wish.

I have explained three clinical observations all of which point to the importance of *amae* as a basic desire. As I said before, the state of *amae* originally refers to what a small child feels toward his mother. It is therefore not surprising that the desire to *amaeru* still influences one's adult years and that it becomes manifest in the therapeutic situation. Here we have a perfect example of transference in the psychoanalytic sense. But then is it not strange that *amaeru* is a unique Japanese word? Indeed, the Japanese find it hard to believe that there is no word for *amaeru* in European languages; a colleague once told me that he could not believe that the equivalent for such a seemingly universal phenomenon as *amae* did not exist in English or German, since, as he put it, 'Even puppies do it, you know.' Let me therefore illustrate the 'Japaneseness' of the concept of *amaeru* by one striking incident. The mother of a Eurasian patient, a British woman who had been a long-term resident of Japan, was discussing her daughter with me. She spoke to me in English, but she suddenly switched to Japanese, in order to tell me that her daughter did not *amaeru* much as a child. I asked her why she had suddenly switched to Japanese. She replied, after a pause, that there was no way to say *amaeru* in English.

I have mentioned two Japanese words that are closely related to the psychology of *amae*: *kodawaru*, which means 'to be inwardly disturbed over one's personal relationships', and *sumanai*, which means 'to feel guilty or obligated'. Now I should like to mention a few more words that are also related to the psychology of *amae*. First, *amai*, which originally means 'sweet', can be used figuratively to describe a person who is overly soft and benevolent toward others or, conversely, one who always expects to *amaeru* in his relationships with others. Second, *amanzuru*, which is derived from *amaeru*, describes the state of mind in which one acquiesces to whatever circumstances one happens to be in. Third, *tori-iru*, which means 'to take in', describes the behavior of a person who skillfully maneuvers another into permitting him to *amaeru*. Fourth, *suneru* describes the behavior of a child or an adult who pouts and sulks because he feels he is not allowed to *amaeru* as much as he wants to, thus harboring in himself mental pain of a masochistic nature. Fifth, *higamu* describes the behavior of a child or an adult who feels himself unfairly treated compared to others who are more favored, often suggesting the presence of a paranoid feeling. Sixth, *tereru* describes the behavior of a child or an adult who is ashamed of showing his intimate wish to *amaeru*. Seventh, *hinekureru* describes the behavior of a child or an adult who takes devious ways in his efforts to deny the wish to *amaeru*.

One could readily say that the behaviors or emotions described by all these Japanese words are not unknown to Westerners and that they appear quite frequently in the therapeutic situation with Western patients. But there remains the question I raised before: Why is there no word in English or in other European languages that is equivalent to *amaeru*, the most central element in all these emotions? To this, one might answer that the absence of a word like *amaeru* is no inconvenience, since it can easily be represented by a combination of words such as the 'wish to be loved' or 'dependency needs'. That may be so, but does not this linguistic difference point to something deeper? Perhaps it reflects a basic psychological difference between Japan and the Western World. Before discussing this problem further, however, I would like to mention a theory of Michael Balint, a British psychoanalyst, which has much bearing on what I am talking about now.

In his psychoanalytic practice Balint observed that 'in the final phase of the treatment patients begin to give expression to long-forgotten, infantile, instinctual wishes, and to demand their gratification from their environment' (Balint, 1952a). He called this infantile desire 'passive object love', since its primal aim is to be loved; he also called it 'primary love', since it is the foundation upon which later forms of love are built. I imagine that he must have wondered why such an important desire is not represented by one common word, for he points out the fact that 'all European languages are so poor that they cannot distinguish between the two kinds of object-love, active and passive' (Balint, 1952b).

By now it must be clear that the 'primary love' or 'passive object-love' described by Balint is none other than the desire to *amaeru*. But then we have to draw the curious conclusion that the emotion of primary love is readily accessible to Japanese patients by way of the word *amaeru*, while to Western patients, according to Balint, it can become accessible only after a painstaking analysis. In my observations I have also noticed that the recognition of *amae* by Japanese patients does not signify the final phase of treatment, as it did in Balint's patients. I think that we have to try to solve this apparent contradiction very carefully, because therein lies, in my opinion, an important key to understanding the psychological differences between Japan and Western countries.

The reasoning behind Balint's observation that primary love appears in its pure form only in the final phase of treatment is as follows: The primary love of an infant is bound to be frustrated, leading to the formation of narcissism; as though he said to himself, 'If the world does not love me enough, I have to love and gratify myself.' Since such narcissism is part of the earliest and most primitive layer of the mind, it can be modified only in the last stage of treatment, at which time the long-repressed urge to be loved can re-emerge in its pure state. Then what shall we say about the Japanese, to whom this primary desire to be loved is always accessible? Does it mean that the Japanese have less narcissism? I think not. Rather I would say that the Japanese somehow continue to cherish the wish to be loved even after the formation of narcissism. It is as though the Japanese did not want to see the reality of their basic frustration. In other words the Japanese, as does everybody else, do experience frustration of their primary love, as is well attested to by the existence of the rich vocabulary we have already encountered relating to the frustration of *amae*. But it seems that the Japanese never give up their basic desire to *amaeru*, thus mitigating the extent of violent emotions caused by its frustration.

In this connection I want to mention an interesting feature of the word *amaeru*. We do not say that an infant does *amaeru* until he is about one year old, thereby indicating that he is then conscious of his wish to *amaeru*, which in turn suggests the presence of a budding realization that his wish cannot always be gratified. Thus, from its inception, the wish to *amaeru* is accompanied by a secret fear that it may be frustrated.

If what I have been saying is true, then it must indicate that there is a social sanction in Japanese society for expressing the wish to *amaeru*. And it must be this social sanction that has encouraged in the Japanese language the development of the large vocabulary relating to *amaeru*. In other words, in Japanese society parental dependency is fostered, and this behavior pattern is even institutionalized into its social structure, whereas perhaps the opposite tendency prevails in Western societies. This seems to be confirmed by recent anthropological studies of Japanese society, notably that of Ruth Benedict, who said: 'The arc of life in Japan is plotted in opposite fashion to that in the United States. It is a great U-curve with maximum freedom and indulgence allowed to babies and to the old. Restrictions are slowly increased after babyhood till having one's own way reaches a low just before and after marriage' (Benedict, 1961). It is true that the restrictions Benedict spoke of do exist for adults in Japanese society, but it should be understood that these restrictions are never meant to be drastic so far as the basic desire to *amaeru* is concerned. Rather, these restrictions are but channels through which that desire is to be duly gratified. That is why we can speak of parental dependency as being institutionalized in Japanese society. For instance, in marriage a husband does *amaeru* toward his wife, and vice versa. It is strongly present in all formal relationships, including those between teacher and student and between doctor and patient. Thus William Caudill (1961), in his observations on Japanese psychiatric hospitals, spoke of the mutual dependency he encountered in all relationships.

In this connection I cannot resist mentioning an episode that happened when I gave a talk on some characteristic Japanese words to a professional group in the United States. *Amaeru* was one of those words. After my talk one distinguished scholar asked me whether or not the feeling of *amaeru* is something like what Catholics feel toward their Holy Mother. Apparently he could not recognize the existence of such a feeling in the ordinary mother-child relationship. And if his response is representative of Americans, it would mean that in American society the feeling of *amaeru* can be indulged in perhaps only in the religious life, but here also very sparingly.

I would now like to mention a study by a Japanese scholar, Hajime Nakamura, professor of Indian philosophy at the University of Tokyo and an authority on comparative philosophy. In his major work, *Ways of Thinking of Eastern Peoples* (1960), he presents a penetrating analysis of thought patterns of Indians, Chinese, Japanese, and Tibetans on the basis of linguistic studies and observations on variations in Buddhist doctrine and practice in these four countries. What he says about the Japanese pattern of thought is parallel to what I have been saying here, though he reaches his conclusions from an entirely different source. He says that the Japanese way of thinking is greatly influenced by an emphasis on immediate personal relations and also that the Japanese have always been eager to adopt foreign cultural influences, but always within the framework of this emphasis on personal relations. To state this in psychoanalytic terms: the Japanese are always prepared to identify themselves with, or introject, an outside force, to the exclusion of other ways of coping with it. This character trait of the Japanese was touched upon by Benedict, too, when she said that 'the Japanese have an ethic of alternatives' and 'Japan's motivations are situational', referring particularly to the sudden complete turnabout of Japan following the defeat of the last war.

This leads, however, to the very interesting and important question of whether or not Japanese character structure has changed at all since the war. I think that Benedict was quite right in assuming that Japan as a whole willingly submitted to unconditional surrender because it was the Emperor's order, that Japan wanted only to please the Emperor, even in her defeat. But it cannot be denied that things have been changing since then. For instance, the Emperor had to declare that he no longer wished to be considered sacred. Also the Japanese have been disillusioned to find that the paramount virtue of *chū*, that is, loyalty to the emperor, was taken advantage of by the ultra-nationalists, who completely failed them. With the decline of *chū* there was also a decline of *kō*, that is, of filial piety. In other words, the tradition of repaying one's *on*, that is, one's spiritual debts to an emperor and to one's parents, was greatly undermined. Thus there developed the moral chaos of present-day Japan.

I think, however, that the nature of this chaos has a distinctly Japanese character and can best be understood by taking into account the psychology of *amae*. It seems that heretofore the stress upon the duty of repaying one's *on* to the emperor and to one's parents served the purpose of regulating the all too powerful desire of *amae*. Since the Japanese were deprived of this regulating force after the war, it was inevitable that their desire to *amaeru* was let loose, with its narcissistic element becoming more manifest. That perhaps explains why we now find in Japan so many examples of lack of social restraint. I wonder whether this recent tendency has also helped to increase the number of neurotics. I think it has, though we have no reliable statistics to confirm it. But I am quite certain that an analysis of the psychology of *amae* such as I am attempting here would not have been possible in prewar days, because *amae* was concealed behind the duty of repaying one's *on*. It certainly was not visible to the outside observer, even to one as acute as Ruth Benedict. I would like to give you one clinical example to illustrate this point.

One of my recent patients, who was a student of law, revealed to me one day his secret thoughts, saying, 'I wish I had some person who would take the responsibility of assisting me.' The remarkable thing about this confession was that the Japanese word that he used for 'assist' was a special legal term *hohitsu*, which was formerly used only for the act of assisting the emperor with his task of governing the nation. In saying this, as the patient himself explained, he wanted, like the emperor, to appear to be responsible for his acts but to depend completely on his assistant, who would really carry the burden. He said this, not jokingly but, rather, with complete seriousness. It is obvious that this confession revealed his secret desire to *amaeru*, about which he spoke more clearly on another occasion. But what I would like to point out here is that in prewar days the patient could hardly have made such a confession, using a special term reserved only for the emperor. Of course, this is a special case, and the fact that the patient was a law student accounted for his use of such a technical term. Yet I think that this case illustrates the point that I want to make, that is, the more emphasis placed upon repaying one's *on*, the less clearly seen is one's desire to *amaeru*.

In this connection, let me say a few words about the nature of so-called 'emperor worship', which served as the Japanese state religion in prewar days. It is true that the emperor was held sacred, but the element of taboo was greater than that of divinity. It is really tempting to apply what Freud said about taboo to the Japanese emperor worship. As a matter of fact, he did mention the Japanese emperor in his book on *Totem and Taboo*, but not from the viewpoint of what is being discussed here. I will not go into this subject any further now, except to add one more comment concerning the effect of elimination of the emperor taboo and its related system, apart from the already discussed release of the desire to *amaeru*. Some Japanese critics voiced the opinion that the tight thought control deriving from the emperor and the family system in prewar days stifled development of healthy selfhood, that one could assert himself in those days only by way of *suneru* and *higamu*, which are interestingly enough the very same Japanese words that I have described before as indicating frustration of *amae* (Maruyama, 1960; Isono, 1960). I agree that this opinion is generally true, but I do not believe that elimination of the emperor and family system alone can lead to development of healthy serfhood or personality. This is shown by many patients, who confess that they are awakened to the fact that they have 'not had self' apart from the all powerful desire to *amaeru*. Then what or who can help them to obtain their 'self'? This touches upon a very important problem of identity, which I will not attempt to discuss in detail. I can say only that the Japanese as a whole are still searching for something, something with which they can safely identify themselves, so that they can become whole, independent beings.

In closing I should like to make two additional remarks. First, it may seem that I am possibly idealizing the West in a way, since I have looked at the problem of personality and culture in modern Japan from the Western point of view. I do not deny that I have. In fact I could not help doing so, because Japanese culture did not produce any yardstick to judge itself critically. I really think that it is a fine thing for the West to have developed such a yardstick for critical analysis. And it seems inevitable that it involves a kind of idealization when the non-Westerners attempt to apply such a yardstick to themselves. I know, however, that in the psychoanalytic circles of Western countries idealization has a special meaning and is not something commendable. So they would certainly not call their use of the analytical method idealization. But I wonder whether they are entirely right in assuming that their use of the analytical method stands on its own without involving any idealization on their part.

Second, though I have stated that there is no exact equivalent to the word *amaeru* in all European languages, I do not say that *amaeru* is unique to the Japanese language. I have some information that the language of Korea and that of Ainu have a word of the same meaning. There seems to be some question about whether or not the Chinese language has such a word. I am now most curious to know whether or not the Polynesian languages have a similar word. I have a feeling that they may have. If they do, how would their psychology compare with that of the Japanese? It is my earnest hope that these questions will he answered by anthropological and psychological studies in the not too distant future.

BIBLIOGRAPHY

BALINT, MICHAEL
1952a 'The Final Goal of Psychoanalytic Treatment'. In *Primary Love and Psychoanalytic Technique*. London: Hogarth Press.
1952b 'Critical Notes on the Theory of the Pregenital Organizations of the Libido'. In: *Ibid.*
BENEDICT, RUTH
1961 *The Chrysanthemum and the Sword*. Boston, Houghton Mifflin Co.
CAUDILL, WILLIAM
1961 'Around the Clock Patient Care in Japanese Psychiatric Hospitals: The Role of the *tsukisoi*', *Amer. Soc. Rev.*, 26:204-14.
DOI, L. TAKEO
1956 'Japanese Language as an Expression of Japanese Psychology', *Western Speech*, 20:90-96.
1958 'Shinkeishitsu no seishinbyori' ('Psychopathology of *shinkeishitsu*'), *Psychiatric et Neurologia Japonica*, 60: 733-44.
1960 'Jibun to amae no seishinbyori' ('Psychopathology of *jibun* and *amae*'), *ibid.*, 61: 149-62.
1961 'Sumanai to Ikenai ("*Sumanai* and *Ikenai*") – Some Thoughts on Super-Ego', *Jap. J. Psychoanal.*, 8:4-7.
ISONO, FUJIKO
1960 'Ie to Jigaishiki' ('Family and Self-consciousness'). In: *Kindai Nippon Shisoshi Kōza* ('History of Thought in Modern Japan'), Vol. 6. Tokyo: Chikuma Shobo.
MARUYAMA, MASAO
1960 *Chūsei to Hangyaku* ('Loyalty and Rebellion'). In: *ibid.*
NAKAMURA HAJIME
1960 *Ways of Thinking of Eastern peoples*. JAPANESE NATIONAL COMMISSION FOR UNESCO (comp.). Tokyo: Japanese Government Printing Bureau.

First published in *Psychologia*, Vol.V, No.3, September 1962. © Psychologia Society, Dept. of Psychology, Kyoto University, Kyoto, Japan

④ Morita Therapy and Psychoanalysis[*]

I am going to attempt here today a comparison between Morita therapy and psychoanalysis. Before doing it, however, a brief exposition of Morita therapy would be required, because I presume this treatment method is not known to you, though in recent years there has been a number of publications, written in English, on this subject and you might have heard of its name. After describing what Morita therapy is like, I will try to interpret Morita therapy in terms of psychoanalytic language. I mean by this an interpretation of the psychodynamics of what takes place in Morita therapy. Then I will speculate on the philosophy behind Morita therapy or rather its cultural background. Lastly, in the light of what we learn about Morita therapy, I will venture to re-examine psychoanalysis and raise a few questions about it.

Morita therapy is so named because its founder is Dr. Shoma Morita,[1] who was professor of psychiatry at Jikei Medical College in Tokyo. It was in the early 1920s that he evolved a special treatment method for a certain kind of neurosis. The types of neurosis he selected for the treatment were neurasthenia, anxiety neurosis and obsessive neurosis, all of which he subsumed under the general category of *shinkeishitsu*, a Japanese word for German *Nervosität*. The reason for his doing so was the following: that all three develop from the common constitution, which he named the 'hypochondriacal constitution'. By using the term 'constitution' he meant the existence of a basic, possibly biologically determined, factor in these neuroses. But by attaching the adjective 'hypochondriacal' to this term he tried to elucidate the psychological aspect of this basic constitution. It is extremely interesting that he took the hypochondriacal state of mind as a very ordinary one, in fact, a very natural human condition. Namely, he stated that this state of mind arises from the fear due to the self-preservative instinct; hence it is universal and exists to a greater or lesser degree in every man. Undoubtedly, the hypochondriacal constitution is the one in which there is a good deal of such an instinctive fear. Morita stops at this point and does not attempt a further analysis of this fear, inasmuch as he takes the hypochondriacal state of mind for granted in the first place. But starting from this seemingly active theory of the hypochondriacal

[*] Presented at N. I. M. H., Bethesda, Maryland, U. S. A., June 11, 1962.

constitution, he constructed further a theory of symptom formation. The hypochondriacal constitution alone does not produce a disease of *shinkeishitsu*. But if one who has such a constitution develops an emotional or autonomous reaction to a certain stimulus and gets caught in such a reaction because of his 'hypochondriacal mood', then it will turn into a permanent symptom, even though otherwise it was only to be a temporary thing. Because, Morita argues, such a reaction will get intensified by the undue attention that was aroused by the hypochondriacal fear, subsequently it will invite more attention to it, and thus set in motion the reciprocal effect of reaction and attention. He called the process of this reciprocal effect *toraware*, a Japanese word which means 'to be caught'. Incidentally, this is a very ordinary Japanese word, and we use it quite often in everyday conversation to express the feeling of being caught or involved or preoccupied. As against this morbid state of mind Morita set forth the ideal state of mind in which one's attention is not unduly arrested by anything and flows smoothly and continuously.

Morita's theory here expounded might look too unsophisticated to those who are immersed in the psychoanalytic sophistication. Without attempting a critical examination of his theory, however, I will now proceed to describe his treatment method. This was developed from his philosophy of psychotherapy that what is most important in treating patients is how to prescribe and administer rest and training according to the need of each individual. For this purpose, he experimented first with keeping a patient or two in his own home. In other words, he practically lived with his patients. Gradually, as the number of patients increased, a part of his house was converted to a hospital ward, and the general scheme of his treatment method became more systematic. It is important to remember here that the Morita hospital was an extension of his home, physically as well as psychologically. Morita specifically called his method of hospital treatment 'the home-like treatment'. This tradition of carrying the home atmosphere into the hospital life has been well kept to this day by his followers.

When Morita finally completed his treatment method, it consisted of four stages, each running for a week or more. In the first stage the patient is put to bed, and is told not to engage in any activity, such as seeing people, talking, reading or smoking, that might divert his attention from his sickness. The physician might come in to see him, but does not talk with him either. This isolation, of course, increases the patient's anxiety, but then the physician tells him not to fight it, just simply to bear it. Morita observed that the patient often experiences a sudden lifting of anxiety only if he stops fighting it. He also believed that this enforced isolation was useful for diagnosis of *shinkeishitsu*, because those of this type could go through this stage and eventually benefit from it, whereas others of different categories could not: for instance, hysterics would act out and schizophrenics would only become worse. After having struggled with his sickness and having become accustomed to his anxiety, the patient would begin to feel bored with staying in bed. When this sign of being bored is detected, the patient is ushered in to the second stage of therapy.

In the second stage the patient is no longer allowed to stay in bed in the daytime, and is encouraged to engage in light manual tasks around the hospital, such as cleaning up the garden, washing the dishes, or working with some material. He is still prohibited from playing or reading or even talking beyond the bare minimum of necessity. Instead he is now asked to write a diary, on which the doctor makes short comments in writing each day. He is also invited to attend informal meetings, usually held in the evening, where he listens to what the physician or some other advanced patients talk about. The main purpose in this second stage is to make the patient aware of his desire for spontaneous activity and also to make him feel the simple joy of doing small things.

When the patient begins to feel like doing heavier work, he moves to the third stage. The emphasis is placed, as in the second stage, on doing things, not on getting some benefit from it. If the patient expresses a concern or worry about doing any specific task, it is pointed out to him, either directly or through comments on his diary, that he is 'being caught' (*toraware*) by such a concern, and he is enjoined to engage in working. His complaints of symptoms, which he is still quite likely to note in his diary and also is allowed to make during informal meetings in the evening, only meet the laconic indifference or scorn of the physician.

Thus, if and after the patient gradually learns that he is able to work and to enjoy doing so, he enters the fourth stage of therapy, which prepares him to get back to the outside life. In this stage the patient is allowed to read only practical material like popular science, history or biography. He still is not allowed to read novels or philosophy; also he is prohibited from concentrating on reading. His daily manual work must come first, and only in short intervals between the tasks is he allowed to read. He also gets the privilege of going out, but only on the pretext of doing errands. By this time he is comfortably enmeshed in interpersonal relations in the hospital, with the staff as well as with the patients. He has learned to be natural and comfortable with himself as he is and with others, a state of mind which often is described by the phrase *aru ga mama*, meaning 'to take things as they are'. This is also the state of mind which Morita described as the ideal, namely the one in which the mind is not unduly arrested by anything and runs smoothly. Reaching this point the patient is discharged.

Now let us proceed to examine what takes place in Morita therapy in terms of the psychodynamics of the patient. I said earlier that Morita established the new diagnostic category of *shinkeishitsu* as an inclusive term for neurasthenia, anxiety neurosis and obsessive neurosis because all these three develop from the common hypochondriacal constitution. It is quite possible to question his reason for doing so, his theory of the hypochondriacal constitution, and also that of symptom-formation. But let us simply follow his intuition that there is something common in these three forms of neurosis in the way they present themselves to the physician. Here comes to our rescue *toraware*, the Japanese word which I explained earlier as meaning 'to be caught', because these patients do seem to be caught in their symptoms, and the Japanese word *toraware* gives a perfect description of such a state of mind. So apart from Morita's theorizing on the state of *toraware* in terms of the so-called reciprocal effect of reaction and attention, we could simply start with the clinical phenomenon of *toraware*.

Here I have to explain to you some of the results of treating those patients of the *shinkeishitsu* type with psychoanalytic treatment.[2] I have observed that they come to develop in the course of treatment almost invariably an enormous sensitivity over what the physician might feel or think about them, with the resulting diminution of their initial state of *toraware*. Then this sensitivity itself could easily be traced back to their hidden wish to be loved, to be taken care of. From repeated observations of such therapeutic processes, I have reached the following formulation over the dynamics of *toraware* in these patients. First, their primary wish to be loved has suffered a critical frustration, possibly in their early life. This leads either to the repression of the wish to be loved and also of the anger due to its frustration, or to their dissociation, which would result in distorted interpersonal relations. Then the feelings accompanying such distorted relations are displaced or introjected as hypochondriacal complaints, thus leading to the end stage of *toraware*. I have been helped in making this formulation by the presence of a unique word in the Japanese vocabulary, *amaeru*, which means 'to depend and presume upon another's love' and 'to indulge in another's kindness'. I say it is a unique word, because there is no single word that corresponds to *amaeru*, so far as I know, in English or any other European language. *Amaeru* usually refers to what a child feels toward his parents, but can be applied to the similar feeling between two adults. I stated in my previous publications that the concept of *amaeru* is technically the same as what Michael Balint[3] called 'passive object love'. He incidentally pointed out that all European languages cannot distinguish between the two kinds of object love, active and passive.

There are a good many things to be said about this interesting word *amaeru* and its concept. Assuming that the desire to be loved which it represents is more primitive and infantile than the desire to love, it is more vulnerable and subject to pathology. Further, assuming that the psychology of *amaeru* is what underlies that of *toraware* in *shinkeishitsu* patients, then this will throw some light on how Morita therapy works with these patients. In Morita therapy, as we saw above, the patient does not primarily aim to acquire an insight; he is only encouraged to reach a certain state of mind after being induced to experience the full effect of *toraware* which he cannot get rid of even if he wishes and tries to do so. His desire of *amaeru* or his dependency wishes may be noticed in passing by the physician, but it never is brought to bear on the patient. Rather, and this is an interesting feature, it seems that the way Morita therapy is conducted curiously circumvents the desire to be loved or to be taken care of on the part of the patient. He is left in isolation, with almost no support, in the first week. His complaints are paid no heed, and he is encouraged to engage only in manual work. True, he is in the hospital with many patients with similar ailments, some of whom may have improved even to his eyes. He also virtually lives with the physician and his assistants, who work along with him and even dine at the same table. These facts undoubtedly give considerable emotional support to the patient, but his hidden warped desire to *amaeru* remains untouched. But I wonder if this kind of technique somehow succeeds in making the patient transcend his pathology in *amaeru*, thus enabling him to recover his normal functioning. This obviously would not be the same as the result gained by psychoanalytic treatment, which laboriously tries to work out the pathology, but it may still be possible to attain the somewhat similar effect simply by its omission.

This is one account of how Morita therapy works in the light of my experiences of treating *shinkeishitsu* patients in psychoanalytic treatment. I do not say that it is the only correct account, nor that the possibilities contained in Morita therapy are exhausted by this account. In this context I would like to say a few words about the possible connection between Morita therapy and Zen Buddhism. It is a known fact that Morita himself not infrequently quoted from old Zen masters for support of his thinking, and recently some of his followers resort mainly to the Zen literature for elucidation of the basic philosophy underlying Morita therapy. But what is really interesting about the possible connection between the two is the fact that, in spite of the obvious similarity between his thinking and Zen Buddhism, Morita disclaimed any special connection between the two. He admitted that he had before exercised himself in Zen practice, but said that he had flunked. It is as though he were to say that having flunked he shed all influences of Zen from himself. In any event, it is known that he had a deep conviction that his theory was based upon a rational scientific thinking, that he twice tried to communicate his thoughts to a German periodical of psychiatry, but each time was turned down on account of its being unintelligible. So it is quite likely that Zen-like thinking slipped against his will into the exposition of his theory, if not into its essence. And it is truly an irony of history that nowadays his theory is associated mostly with Zen Buddhism in the minds of Western scholars.

In my opinion, what definitely links Morita theory to Zen Buddhism is its conception of the ideal state of mind as the one in which the mind is not unduly arrested by anything and flows smoothly and continuously. In Morita therapy the patient is told not to shy away from his feelings, rather to accept them. Then this would not look different from what is set forth as the ideal in psychoanalytic treatment. But in the case of Morita therapy there seems to be a slight element of detachment in the way one accepts one's feelings. This is partly because in Morita therapy one does not go out to probe one's feelings as one does in psychoanalysis, rather one is encouraged to look at them summarily as things that simply happen; partly because one is practically made to stand aloof from the conflict-ridden self by engaging his whole person in manual work. As I mentioned earlier, Morita therapy does not aim at exploration of one's pathology, but I wonder if it also evades or perhaps transcends an issue of great importance by overpassing the pathology. In saying this I have in mind one interesting clinical phenomenon which one can observe in psychoanalytic treatment of *shinkeishitsu* patients. They would almost invariably experience a painful sense of 'not-having-possessed-their-selves-before' after they become aware of their hidden wish to *amaeru*. But this kind of experience will not occur to patients in Morita therapy, because here one is helped to attain a state of mind in which one is even forgetful of oneself. Truly this is related to the Zen ideal of no self. Since the perception of one's individual separate self is most disturbing, it has to be dissolved in the feeling of unity with one's surroundings or with nature. Perhaps I should say 'with Mother Nature', which is more meaningful psychoanalytically.

I would now like to look at this characteristic of Morita therapy again from a different angle. I think that the experience one is supposed to get in Morita therapy has almost an aesthetic quality. It certainly is not moralistic in spite of its confining the patients to the home-like hospital life and also its emphasis on manual work. The element of detachment from one's conflict-ridden life, which I spoke of a while ago, is undoubtedly congenial with aesthetic life. Even the emphasis on manual work is, as was explained before, not for any utilitarian purpose. Morita is said to have told patients, 'Do lose yourself in whatever work you do.' 'Lose yourself' is a poor translation of his original words. They are literally 'do become the act of doing anything you do'. This, of course, does not exclude the genuine pleasure of work, rather it is meant to enhance it; hence it is tantamount to converting housework or any chore into artistic engagement. Thus this preponderance of aesthetic or artistic elements in Morita therapy fits in very well with Japanese culture in which it was born, since, as you probably know, or rather as I see it, the best quality of Japanese culture lies in her aesthetics and arts.

Now finally we come back to the task of examining psychoanalysis in the light of what we have learned about Morita therapy. Curiously enough, a very strange image of psychoanalysis emerges from the perspective of Morita therapy; that the former is terribly moralistic treatment compared with the latter, in spite of the often-raised criticisms in Western societies that psychoanalysis is antimoral, or at least amoral. I here use the adjective 'moralistic' not pejoratively, but then I have to qualify what I mean by this. For this purpose let me choose two problems of authority and dependency among others and see how they are dealt with in psychoanalysis. First, speaking of the problem of authority, one would almost automatically think that Morita therapy is authoritarian, while psychoanalysis is individualistic. I do not necessarily deny the validity of such a description, if one is to be satisfied by surface phenomena. But if one looks deeper, an entirely different picture comes to our view. Certainly in Morita therapy hospitals the patients would take deep bows to their physician and would not think of saying anything critical about him. So one may say that the authoritarian atmosphere prevails in Morita therapy hospitals. But what can one say about the fact that Morita therapists work together with the patients and dine with them? They often even tell the patients that they have suffered from the same problem as the patients now do. So the prevailing atmosphere in Morita therapy hospitals is most congenial and warm in spite of the patients' due respect toward the physician. In contrast with Morita therapy, in psychoanalysis the patient faces his therapist as his equal. He certainly would not take deep bows to the therapist. He is even encouraged to say anything critical or negative about the therapist. He is free either to continue or discontinue therapy. But it is illusory to deduce from this apparent use of freedom that psychoanalysis is devoid of any function of authority. On the contrary, Freud himself stated that 'Analysis . . . presupposes the consent of the analysed; the situation of analysis involves a superior and a subordinate.'[4] This is not to negate the freedom of patients, certainly not to impose any moral demand on the patient, as Freud specifically stated to that effect elsewhere. But one has to be reminded that it takes perhaps even a greater authority to tell another human being, in this case a patient, that he is free to do whatever he chooses with his life. Furthermore, in psychoanalysis one is not even promised one's eventual cure, yet one would be ready to remain in therapy for an indefinite length of time. I wonder what would be authority if this kind of commitment does not presuppose the existence of authority, even though it may not be so named and recognized as such.

Speaking of the matter of length of treatment leads to another problem of dependency which I chose for discussion. The length of Morita therapy is comparatively short, at most runs to only a few months, while the length of psychoanalytic treatment is by nature indefinite. It is true that in the case of Morita therapy the patients do often keep contact with the physician even after their discharge, that at times they even form a group of ex-patients. But, as I said earlier, it is not in the nature of Morita therapy to deal with the patient's dependency wishes, rather it bypasses or possibly transcends them, whereas in psychoanalysis one has to labor with one's dependency wishes, has to probe every aspect of them; curiously enough, however, for that purpose one is allowed to depend upon one's analyst. But then one is required constantly to examine one's dependency on the analyst, eventually to save the golden core from the crude ore for future reference. I think this difference between Morita therapy and psycho-analysis in terms of their attitude toward dependency is a reflection of different characteristics of Japanese society and Western societies. In

Japanese society there are so many channels in which one can easily gratify one's dependency wishes. Only if one can transcend one's petty conflicts over dependency can one easily be integrated into the society. But in Western societies the requirement for an individual seems to be nominally high. Unless one becomes truly independent, one cannot satisfactorily function in those societies. Hence one would have to undergo a longer period of re-education or longer apprenticeship, which is what psychoanalysis certainly looks like to the Japanese in comparison with Morita therapy.

I have been allowing myself to speculate on the cross-cultural differences between Japanese and Western societies. In comparing Morita therapy and psychoanalysis, one eventually has to come up with the problem of a more basic difference between the two cultures in which these treatment methods were born. Not being trained in anthropology and cultural studies, I shall no more be able to enlarge on this subject, but in order to further your thinking on the effect of culture on treatment method let me call your attention lastly to the following fact. There is good evidence to believe that Morita himself suffered from the illness of *shinkeishitsu*, and so did many of his followers. One may almost be justified to say that in the last analysis he evolved his treatment method out of his own struggles with his illness. Now interestingly enough, one can't help feeling from reading Freud's biography that he himself suffered from *shinkeishitsu* – I mean his hypochondriacal symptoms, anxiety attacks, and hidden mother attachment. But it seems that he approached this problem from an entirely different angle from that of Morita. As we all know, he tried to understand this in terms of sexual economy. To take the hypochondriacal state of mind as something ordinary, almost self-explanatory, did not occur to Freud as it did so naturally to Morita. Why is this difference? If this question is meaningful, we are again thrown back on cultural differences between the two. I know Freud vigorously objected to the interpretation of his theory in terms of his personality and culture. But I don't think Morita would have objected so much to a similar attempt. Again, why is this difference?

So this is my story of a comparison between Morita therapy and psychoanalysis. I do not deny that I have oversimplified both for the sake of argument. But I shall be very happy indeed if my story aroused a new curiosity about something you thought you were familiar with, and at least provoked you to some further thinking.

NOTES

1. Morita, Shoma. *Shinkeishitsu ito hontai to ryoho* (Essence and treatment of *shinkeishitsu*). 1928. (New edition, with commentary by Hiroshi Kawai, published by Hakuyosha, Tokyo, in 1960).
2. Doi, Takeo. *Shinkeishitsu no seishinbyori* (Psychopathology of *shinkeishitsu*). *Seishin-*

Shinkeigaku Zasshi (Psychiatria et Neurologia Japonica), 1958, 60, 733-744.

3. Balint, Michael. *Primary love and psychoanalytic technique.* London: Hogarth Press, 1956. (See also: *Amae* – A key concept for understanding Japanese personality structure. *Psychologica*, 1962, 5, 1-7.)

4. Freud, Sigmund. *On the history of the psychoanalytic movement.* Collected Papers, Vol. 1. London: Hogarth Press, 1950.

First published in Psychiatry. *Journal for the Study of Interpersonal Processes.* Vol.26, No.3, August 1963. © The William Alanson White Psychiatric Foundation, Inc.

⑤ Some Thoughts on Helplessness and the Desire To Be Loved*

The title of this paper may seem, to the speaker of English or any European language, to refer to two quite distinct ideas which have no necessary relationship. I am attempting, however, in this title to convey the main elements of what is a single concept in the Japanese language and culture, expressed most specifically in the verb *amaeru*, although there are other words which express variations on this theme. I have chosen this as the subject of this paper for two reasons. First, in my clinical work in Japan I have found that this concept is very useful in formulating the psychodynamics of neurotic patients. Furthermore, it seems to be useful for understanding the cultural context of Japanese society as well. Second, I think that what can be said about this concept may have a broader implication beyond the mere description of the regional characteristics of Japanese patients or society. In other words, although there is no single term in English which expresses this concept, I doubt that the underlying psychology is alien to English-speaking peoples, and I believe that this concept may serve as a kind of corrective for a certain type of thinking which is prevalent in American psychiatry.

In working with neurotic patients in Japan,[1] my attention was called to the singular phenomenon that these patients almost invariably present themselves as quite helpless, a feeling which usually becomes intensified in the course of treatment, along with the development of a hypersensitivity about what the therapist might feel or think about them. One might say that the patient develops such a sensitivity toward the therapist because the therapeutic situation promises help but does not at once give him the kind of help he wants. I subsequently realized that his initial helplessness and subsequent sensitivity really refer to the wish to be loved or to be taken care of. I was helped in detecting this wish by recalling the meaning of the intransitive verb *amaeru*, which may be translated as 'to depend and presume upon another's love' or 'to indulge in another's kindness'. Many patients actually used the verb *amaeru*, either describing the frustration of the wish in their interpersonal relationships or indicating the wish at the

* This paper has been presented at the Washington School of Psychiatry, at the University of Pittsburgh, and at Yale Unlversity.

31

height of the transference.

The clinical facts seemed to suggest the following formulation regarding the psychodynamics of these patients: their primary wish to be loved had suffered a critical frustration, probably in early life. This, however, did not necessarily lead to the repression of the wish to be loved. Instead, it seemed that the anger or direct hostility due to the frustration was usually repressed in the service of keeping the original wish to be loved alive.

Yet the early frustration led to manifold distortions of the wish and to a continuing fear of further frustration. The symptoms of various kinds could then be interpreted as the intrapsychic working-over of early traumatic experiences.[2]

I have become convinced from my clinical experience in Japan as well as in the United States that the warped desire to be loved and cared for plays a central role in all kinds of psychopathology. But uncovering this desire is probably easier with Japanese neurotic patients than with such patients from other cultures. At this point I can almost anticipate an admonition to the effect that I am possibly making too much of dependency phenomena which are commonplace in patients, that I am making a mountain out of a molehill. I concede that such phenomena are commonplace, but I do not think it necessarily follows that they are unimportant. Further, the reason why I can make a mountain out of a molehill, if I do, is that there is such a convenient word as *amaeru* in the Japanese language, which facilitates a meaningful interpretation of what it expresses.[3]

This word, to explain its connotations further, usually describes what a small child feels toward his parents, particularly his mother, or his behavior indicating the presence of such a feeling. Hence it covers the wish to be taken care of or the wish to cling to the love object. The word derives from *amai*, meaning 'sweet', and it suggests infantile dependency. In this connection, however, one might argue that a small child can be conscious of a wish to be taken care of, or for warm contact, but cannot be so directly conscious of a wish to be loved, which belongs to adult psychology. Certainly in English phrasing these seem like somewhat different wishes, but the beauty of the Japanese word *amaeru* is that it can suggest the common origin of all these wishes as stemming from the early years of life. In fact, even though the word clearly evokes feelings pertaining to childhood, it is just as often used to describe similar feelings or behavior that occur between two adults, such as husband and wife, master and subordinate, or teacher and student. Such usage of the word seems very reasonable indeed, because there is no reason why a mode of behavior developed in the early years of life has to be confined to that period alone. Thus the childlike flavor of the word is helpful in isolating and tracing the feelings which it expresses of helplessness and the desire to be loved.

I think that this unique feature of the Japanese language must reflect certain characteristics of Japanese society. It certainly seems to bespeak the fact that in Japan dependency upon the parents is fostered and institutionalized into the social structure. Japanese society has been studied by many scholars in recent years, but I believe that most of them have not taken sufficiently into account the psychological importance of dependency on the parents or the continuing importance of the originally infantile wish to be loved. There are a few exceptions, however; Ezra Vogel has confirmed by his observations the fostering of dependency in child-rearing in Japan,[4] and William Caudill has pointed out the dominant pattern of dependent relationships in his observations of psychiatric hospital patients and personnel in Japan.[5] Caudill has now begun to study mother-child interaction in Japan, and from his pilot study[6] I will single out the following finding for its relevance to the present theme. He observed that Japanese mothers are in almost constant attendance on their babies and are likely to pick them up or otherwise divert them as soon as they cry. If this observation can be trusted, and I think it can, it bears out my own observation of the notion Japanese mothers seem to have of their babies – that they are essentially helpless. In my opinion, this differs decisively from the common Western notion that babies are inherently autonomous, and the more autonomous they become, the better.[7] It seems likely that the kind of child-rearing based mainly on the former idea will nurture and perpetuate the state of helplessness or the wish to be loved, thus leading to the formation of a social structure that takes care of such a need.

It was for this reason that I said earlier that the analysis of the wish to be loved would probably be easier with Japanese patients than with Western patients. Certainly the rich vocabulary regarding the psychology of *amaeru* and the social sanction for it would make it easier for Japanese patients to become aware of their wish to be loved and to express it. Not only patients, but ordinary adults can allow themselves to indulge in the feeling of helplessness at times. This does not necessarily mean that dependency wishes are always truly gratified in Japan, although one could perhaps gratify one's dependency wishes to a greater extent in Japan than in the United States. On the contrary, the existence of the rich vocabulary regarding the psychology of *amaeru* and the social sanction for it could indicate a preoccupation with the wish to be loved, which might have been born out of a dire necessity to deal with this vital wish. In other words, for the Japanese mind, to be helpless is a basic fact of human existence that cannot be eliminated or resolved. What one can do for helpless beings then is, in essence, to have pity or sympathy for them, or, to put it in psychoanalytic terms, to identify oneself with their helplessness. I think that this is the Japanese notion of love or affection, and that it was reinforced and cultivated for centuries by Buddhism, if not originated by it.

So far, I have tried to show that the concept of helplessness and the desire to be loved supplies an important key for the interpretation of Japanese psychiatric and cultural material. Now I would like to turn to theoretical considerations. I have already indicated that this concept refers primarily to the phenomena of the early years of life, the most important phase of human development. So far as psychoanalytic literature is concerned, this concept has not received primary consideration but instead seems to have been subsumed under the more hypothetical concepts of narcissism and omnipotence. In saying this, I am not unaware of the fact that Freud himself discussed the tender, affectionate feelings of a child[8] and his fear of separation from his mother[9] or the fact that in recent years increasing attention has been focused on the aspect of mother-transference in the therapeutic situation.[10] But it seems to me that, theoretically speaking, the concepts of narcissism and omnipotence have become 'overvalued' ideas for most analysts, except for Michael Balint, whom I will discuss later. To clarify my point, let me quote what Freud said about these two concepts:

> The primary narcissism of children which we have assumed and which forms one of the postulates of our theories of the libido, is less easy to grasp by direct observation than to confirm by inference from elsewhere. If we look at the attitude of affectionate parents towards their children, we have to recognize that it is a revival and reproduction of their own narcissism, which they have long since abandoned.[11]

> . . . *loving oneself* . . . we regard as the characteristic feature of narcissism. Then, according as the object or the subject is replaced by an extraneous one, what results is the active aim of loving or the passive one of being loved – the latter remaining near to narcissism.[12]

> We speak of the narcissism of small children, and it is to the excessive narcissism of primitive man that we ascribe his belief in the omnipotence of his thoughts and his consequent attempts to influence the course of events in the external world by the technique of magic.[13]

The question I raise here is why it is necessary to set up these overriding concepts of primary narcissism and omnipotence for the facts of helplessness and the wish to be loved. I do not think that Freud is convincing when he says that primary narcissism, which he admits is an assumption, can be confirmed by inference from the attitude of affectionate parents, because it can be perceived as 'a revival and reproduction of their own narcissism, which they have long since abandoned'. It seems to me much simpler and more reasonable to think of the attitude of affectionate parents as a revival and reproduction of their own still continuing desire to be loved and cared for, rather than to derive this desire from the hypothetical concept of primary narcissism. There appears to be no good theoretical reason for this derivation, except, perhaps, the necessity of depositing libido somewhere. As for the concept of omnipotence, I admit that this may be a good descriptive term, although a bit too fanciful, for a certain pathological or primitive state of mind. But the trouble is that this originally descriptive term was elevated to become an explanatory concept like the concept of narcissism, and I cannot help feeling that even its descriptive use is a little comical in effect, if not derisive, because in all cases of so-called 'omnipotence' of thought the person is known to be really fearful and extremely helpless.

I will not further complain about the concepts of primary narcissism and omnipotence, since my aim is not to discuss them as such. Before leaving this subject, however, I wish to indicate that my views are close to those of Michael Balint.[14] He has dispensed with the concept of primary narcissism and installed as basic the desire to be loved, which he calls passive object love and to which he attributes the development of narcissism. As for the concept of omnipotence, he states:

> I am afraid it is another example of our thinking in adultomorph language. In fact, 'omnipotence' never means a real feeling of power; on the contrary, a desperate and very precarious attempt at overcoming a feeling of helplessness and impotence.[15]

The question I would like to raise is why Balint alone comes to this conclusion, while most followers of Freud share his view regarding the concepts of narcissism and omnipotence without questioning them. One could, in fact, ask why Freud arrived at these concepts in the first place, if they are not adequately accounted for theoretically. Biographical evidence suggests that he had a serious conflict about the desire to be loved and about seeking help,[16] and thus he might have had to explain away these states of mind intellectually. But I suspect that it is less Freud's personal problems that are responsible for these concepts of narcissism and omnipotence than the cultural heritage which he shared with many of his contemporaries of modern Western civilization.

In order to make clear my view on this question, I think it pertinent to refer to Freud's celebrated essay, 'The Future of an Illusion', in which he dealt with the problem of religion mainly from the viewpoint of human helplessness. In fact, it seems to me that 'Some Thoughts on Helplessness' would have been an equally fitting title, if not more so. Now, his line of reasoning was as follows: Religion is an illusion, because it is based on wishful thinking and converts helplessness into an unrealistic belief that one is taken care of by a beneficent Providence. On the contrary, sensible people 'will have to admit to themselves the full extent of their helplessness and their insignificance in the machinery of the universe. . . . They will be in the same position as a child who has left the parental house where he was so warm and comfortable. But surely infantilism is destined to be surmounted.'[17]

It is not my intention here to defend religion by refuting Freud's reasoning, but I would like to question the implication that religion always converts helplessness into a comfortable belief. Religion does not blot out the feeling of helplessness; rather, in authentic religious experiences, one is likely to feel more intensely helpless. For instance, the whole edifice of Buddhism seems to rest on the recognition of human helplessness and on human compassion for it. Even in Christianity, although one would find comfort in a beneficent Providence, at the same time one must have 'fear and trembling', as Kierkegaard so poignantly argued, and would never think of attributing 'omnipotence' to one's thoughts. I think that the feeling of helplessness is more likely to be blotted out or perhaps repressed among those who consider that they are supposed to grow out of this sign of 'infantilism' and that they have to help themselves.

I believe that you will unmistakably notice in this latter position the cultural norm of man's autonomy or self-help which has been a guiding principle in modern Western civilization. One can say that Freud's essay on 'The Future of an Illusion' was, after all, a psychological interpretation of this norm, demonstrating once again that he was a child of his age and culture. Yet it must be remembered that the naïve optimism of Western man regarding his civilization was gradually declining at the time when Freud wrote this essay. Pertinently, he was reported to have commented later on this essay: 'Now it already seems childish; fundamentally I think otherwise; I regard it as weak analytically and inadequate as a self confession.'[18] He was clearly dissatisfied with what he had written, but unfortunately did not specify in what way it was inadequate and what his real thoughts were. So I will venture to advance my own interpretation. I think that what he wrote was analytically weak and inadequate as a self-confession because the philosophy he seemed to espouse did not provide a useful theoretical framework for analytical therapy and also because his sense of helplessness was still too keen to be replaced by a belief in the progress of science, including his own contribution of psychoanalysis. In this respect one could perhaps refer to his sustained interest in occultism.

I would like to elaborate further on the point that the philosophy of self-help, as it is understood today, is entirely a Western product. Although I am not a historian, I believe that the idea of self-help or the intrinsic autonomy of a person gradually became popular in Western Europe during the early Renaissance. One may perhaps associate the development of this idea with the saying, 'God helps those who help themselves', which seems to have become popular by the seventeenth century. It was used by Algernon Sidney in his political essay, *Discourses Concerning Government*, written around 1680,[19] and a similar saying appears in George Herbert's *Outlandish Proverbs*, first published in 1640.[20] Interestingly enough, this saying in another form can be found in old Greek authors, but not in authentic Judeo-Christian literature, including the Bible. One might well argue, then, that the 'God' of 'God helps those who help themselves', who does not take the initiative in helping people, but only waits for them to help themselves, is not a Judeo-Christian God. Incidentally, such an interpretation is quite possible from Sidney's book, since he uses the saying primarily to point to the grim, almost cruel reality of the hostile world, and scarcely to a helping God. Such a God can easily be dispensed with, because He cannot be depended upon, and what counts, after all, is whether one helps oneself or not. I think that this is what has really happened in modern Western civilization, along with the development of the ideal of self-help or self-determination as a central theme in many competing ideologies.

While I have, of course, been indulging in speculation which might best be left to specialists in the history of civilization, the reason I have done so is that the ideal of self-help invoked by Freud as a philosophy to cope with human helplessness is, in my opinion, a poor working principle for analytic therapy. In psychotherapy the patient is primarily helpless, and that is why he seeks help. But if the therapist meets the patient with the notion that his own function is to help the patient if he helps himself, does this not unduly enhance the patient's feeling of helplessness? Obviously, he would not have sought therapy in the first place if he could help himself. I think that such a situation constitutes a classic example of what Gregory Bateson calls the double bind.[21] It would deeply perplex the patient and only entangle him in an intricate net of transference and countertransference.

While it would be an exaggeration to say that most psychotherapies conducted in the United States are like this, I cannot help feeling that a great many psychotherapists are curiously blind to the possible existence of such a double bind. I have observed on many occasions that patients are left to stew in helplessness simply because they are supposed to help themselves – that is, because of the cultural norm of self-help which is shared by patient and therapist alike. The patient's helplessness tends either to be ignored, or, if noticed, to be treated only as such – in other words, his underlying dependency wishes are not usually taken up.

In order to forestall misunderstanding, however, let me say at once that I am not suggesting going to the other extreme of helping the patient by all means and in whatever ways he wishes to be helped. I am also not negating the ideal of self-help or independence as a goal of psychotherapy. I am only objecting to the cultural assumption which many psychotherapists in this country seem to share unwittingly that they can help the patient only insofar as he helps himself. I think that the process of psychotherapy has to be defined differently: namely, the psychotherapist helps the patient so that he will eventually be able to help himself. Only within this framework, I believe, can that vicious double bind I spoke of be eliminated, and the psychotherapist become capable of appreciating the patient's helplessness and acknowledging his desire to be loved without rejection or compromise, thus making it possible to analyze his pathology in terms of this basic desire to be loved.

You have probably noticed that I have now come full circle and arrived at my point of departure. To use a Chinese expression, it may be said that I am 'drawing the water to my own rice field'. But let me make it clear that I am not claiming that Japanese society provides the best climate for psychotherapy because it fosters dependency and supports the feeling of helplessness. On the contrary, psychoanalysis or any other individual psychotherapy has not yet seen its day in Japan. And I think that the reason is because we have had no ideal of self-help in our tradition. Indeed, we have a popular deity in our mythology who flew into an extreme oral rage because he lost his mother and could not bear the grief. We have had no conception of a God who is self-sufficient, omnipotent, and helpful to human beings, and this leads me to speculate that such a conception might, after all, have been necessary for the development of psychotherapy in Western civilization, particularly in order to strengthen the identity of the psychotherapist. I say this at the risk of investing the psychotherapist with omnipotence. I think that the fact that he has constantly to fight against the illusion of omnipotence in his practice does not necessarily disprove my proposition. If anything, it rather proves it. This, of course, is only my conjecture, but I hope that it may provoke further thinking.

NOTES

1.   L. Takeo Doi 'Psychopathology of *Shinkeishitsu*', *Psychiat. et Neur. Jap.* (1958) 60:733-744.
2.   While this formulation is, of course, an over-simplification of a more complicated neurotic process, It is specifically applicable to the very common neurosis in Japan called *shinkeishitsu*, the Japanese term for the German *Nervosität*. According to Shōma Morita, who first used this word as a diagnostic term, it includes neurasthenia, anxiety neurosis, and a certain form of obsessive neurosis: the patient comes, however, with a hypochondriacal preoccupation, apparently seeking medical help. The analysis of this preoccupation uncovers both his helplessness and his desire to be loved, and shows that he actually is soliciting sympathy and care.
3.   L. Takeo Doi. '*Amae* – A Key Concept for Understanding Japanese Personality Structure', *Psychologia* (1962) 5:1-7.
4.   Ezra Vogel, 'Child Rearing', Chapter 12 from an unpublished book manuscript, *Japan's New Middle Class: The Salary Man and his Family in a Tokyo Suburb*.
5.   William Caudill and L. Takeo Doi, 'Interrelations of Psychiatry, Culture, and Emotion in Japan', in *Medicine and Anthropology*, edited by Iago Galdston; New York, Internat. Univ. Press, 1963.
6.   William Caudill, 'Maternal Care and Infant Behavior in Japan', unpublished manuscript.
7.   Of course, different Western mothers differ somewhat in their attitudes, and of late many of them have been influenced toward a more permissive attitude in regard to their infants by psychodynamicists who believe that this fosters the feeling of being loved which leads to mental health. Yet the mother who dotes on her infant upon expert advice is doing so by calculation rather than instinctively, and her fostering of her child's dependency certainly does not extend beyond the nursing period, as in the Japanese case.
8.   Sigmund Freud, 'On the Universal Tendency to Debasement In the Sphere of Love', *Standard Edition of the Complete Psychological Works* 11:170-190; London, Hogarth, 1957; p. 180.
9.   Sigmund Freud, 'Inhibitions, Symptoms and Anxiety', *Standard Edition of the Complete Psychological Works* 20:75-175; London, Hogarth, 1959.
10   See, for example, John Bowlby, 'The Nature of the Child's Tie to His Mother', *Internat. J. Psychoanalysis* (1958) 39:350-373.
11.   Sigmund Freud, 'On Narcissism: An Introduction', *Standard Edition of the Complete Psychological Works* 14:73-102; London, Hogarth, 1957; pp. 90-91.
12.   Sigmund Freud. 'Instincts and Their Vicissitudes', *Standard Edition of the Complete Psychological Works* 14:117-140; London, Hogarth, 1957; p. 133.
13.   Sigmund Freud, 'A Difficulty In the Path of Psycho-Analysis'. *Standard Edition of the Complete Psychological Works* 17.137-143; London, Hogarth, 1955; p. 139.
14.   Michael Balint, 'Critical Notes on the Theory of the Pregenital Organizations of the

Libido', Chapter 3, in *Primary Love and Psychoanalytic Technique*; London, Hogarth, 1952.

15. Michael Balint, 'On Love and Hate', Chapter 8, in *Primary Love and Psychoanalytic Technique*; London, Hogarth, 1952; p. 145.

16. Ernest Jones. *The Life and Work of Sigmund Freud*, Vols. I and II; New York, Basic Books, 1953, 1955: see Vol. I, pp. 122, 129, 189, and Vol. II, pp. 176, 420.

17. Sigmund Freud, 'The Future of an Illusion'. *Standard Edition of the Complete Psychological Works* 21:5-56; London, Hogarth, 1961; p. 49.

18. Freud, quoted in Ernest Jones, *The Life and Work of Sigmund Freud*, Vol. IV; New York, Basic Books, 1957; p. 138.

19. Algernon Sidney, *Discourses Concerning Government*; London. J. Littlebury, 1698. See also Bartlett's *Familiar Quotations* (13th ed.); New York, Little, Brown, 1955.

20. George Herbert, *Outlandish Proverbs*; London, J. C. Hotten, 1874.

21. Gregory Bateson, Don D. Jackson, Jay Haley, and John Weakland, 'Toward a Theory of Schizophrenia', *Behavioral Science* (1956) 1:251-264.

First published in *The International Journal of Psychiatry*, Congress Issue, 1964

⑥ Psychoanalytic Therapy and 'Western Man': A Japanese View

It is generally believed that theoretically psychoanalytic therapy should be applicable irrespective of cultural differences, because it is based upon the scientific knowledge of the human mind. Freud himself stated as follows: 'I have been able to help people with whom I had nothing in common, neither nationality, education, social position nor outlook upon life in general.'[1] This orientation of psychoanalytic therapy, I think, does imply two things. First, what one values in life, whether it is material or spiritual, is to be analyzed in terms of man's basic needs. Second, in psychoanalytic therapy all value judgments are withheld, hence it does not interfere with one's cultural and moral values, rather respects one's independent judgment and freedom in this area. In other words, even though psychoanalytic therapy subjects all of the patient's values to analysis and neither exhorts nor condemns him, it none the less lives by one supreme value, the respect for his potential independence and basic freedom. In this sense it definitely cannot be thought of as a merely technical device for therapeutic purpose. It may be said that it carries a cultural value within its very technique.

This cultural aspect of psychoanalytic therapy dawned on Western analysts in recent years when it was found that the practice of psychoanalytic therapy became virtually impossible under totalitarian governments which attempt to regiment people, mind and body, completely. In my opinion, the fate of psychoanalytic therapy in Japan is a case of a different kind that also suggests a possible connection between psychoanalytic therapy and the social condition. Psychoanalysis was first introduced into Japan as early as 1912. Since then there has been a steady increase of psychoanalytic literature. In 1918 a professor of psychiatry at one of the national universities started a course in psychoanalytic psychiatry. His student, Dr. Kosawa, went to Vienna in 1931 for psychoanalytic training and subsequently opened the first psychoanalytic clinic in Tokyo. Around 1930 all the main works of Freud had been translated into Japanese. Notwithstanding this early start of the psychoanalytic movement and the absence of violent opposition to psychoanalysis in Japan, the influence of psychoanalysis scarcely reached beyond a small circle of interested people to the main bulk of Japanese psychiatrists, let alone the general populace. Perhaps one reason for this was the fact that Japanese psychiatry was under the heavy influence of German psychiatry, which was almost totally deaf to psychoanalysis at that time. But it alone cannot explain what happened and one gets an impression that Japanese culture and society lacked that certain quality which favors the practice of psychoanalytic therapy.

Let me elucidate then the seeming incompatibility of Japanese culture with psychoanalytic therapy in the light of the latter's cultural aspect as was mentioned above. As for the model of Japanese personality structure, I have written elsewhere.[2] To summarize my argument here, in Japan the dependency of children on parents is fostered even beyond the nursing period and its behavior pattern is institutionalized into its social structure. One telling evidence of this fact is given in a unique Japanese word, *amaeru*, a very common intransitive verb meaning 'to depend and presume upon another's love' and 'to bask in another's indulgence'. It usually refers to what a child feels or what his behavior indicates that he feels toward his parents. But it also can be applied to similar feelings between two adults. In fact, it may be said that all interpersonal relationships in Japan are tinged with the feeling of *amaeru* on the part of both partners, either overtly or covertly. The following two popular sayings illustrate this point: 'Go under a big tree, if you want to depend', 'A nail that sticks out will be hit hard'. The first one recommends dependency and the second prohibits independence. It is clear that such a social climate presents the psychoanalyst with a very difficult task of treating the patient's dependency wish. Because, in the first place, it makes it particularly hard for the analyst to become independent in order to maintain the detached neutral attitude required for analysis; and, in the second place, even if he overcame his own difficulty, he then cannot proceed on the assumption that his respect for individual independence and freedom will be appreciated by the patient.

In Western society, too, the patient of course is dependent upon the therapist. But it always has been supposed that the patient's dependency is transitory and it will go away once the patient solves his problems. Thus the psychology of dependency has rarely been subjected to analytical probing as infantile sexuality has. Freud was not unaware, however, of the importance of dependency. It can be seen in his discussion of religion as a panacea for human helplessness.[3] But apart from his thesis this discussion seems to suggest a cultural bias peculiar to Western society that religion is the main thing that takes care of man's dependency wish, since the latter cannot be satisfied in the ordinary human relationships. I should think in this regard that what he named 'oceanic feeling' was also conceptually related to dependency, since it is defined as the feeling of being inseparably united with the universe.[4] Freud, interestingly enough, disavowed such a feeling to himself and though he used this concept for a critical analysis of religious psychology, he never applied it to clinical phenomena in general. It was Michael Balint among orthodox analysts, so far as I know, who first recognized the immense importance of dependency in individual psychopathology. He described various manifestations of dependency in analysis and arrived at the concept of passive object love as the most primary wish of man.[5] This concept, it seems to me, precisely denotes the wish to *amaeru*. But contrary to my experience with Japanese patients, Balint observed that such a wish would be expressed in its unadulterated form only in the final phase of psychoanalytic therapy.[6] I think this difference must come from the fact that in Japanese society the expression of dependency wish is expected and is responded, whereas in Western society it is discouraged unless it is couched in religious terms.

Significantly, in accordance with the difference in treatment of dependency wish between Japanese and Western society, Japanese has the word *amaeru* and European languages have no equivalent verb to express dependency wish. Balint specifically states that all European languages are so poor that they cannot distinguish between the two kinds of object love, active and passive.[7] How should we account for this phenomenon in psychoanalytic terms? The dependency wish as expressed by *amaeru* may be defined as 'to seek a restoration of the once lost quasi-union of mother and infant' or, borrowing Freud's term, 'to seek to experience the oceanic feeling'. It at once attempts to overcome the pain of separation and to deny its reality. In other words, it can be said that one who does *amaeru* presumes upon the oneness of self and other. For the average person in Japanese society, however, the oneness of self and other is usually only a pretension or at most an illusion shared by the majority of one's group. But some people may be driven to a profound negation, as in Zen Buddhism where one's self is submerged into a Cosmic Self and the identity of subject and object is intuited. I cannot judge how valid and meaningful such an experience really is. At any rate, the emphasis is on an immediate experience as it is actually felt. In contrast with this trend, in Western society the boundary of one's self has always been jealously guarded, and the dichotomy of subject and object has weighed heavily upon one's inner consciousness. Hence, the right and the independence of an individual are stressed and one is prevented from taking recourse to a word like *amaeru* in order to express one's deeply buried need.

It is a known fact that the conflicts over libidinal or aggressive impulses become acute only when the boundary between self and other is established. Accordingly, dependence will alleviate or cover up those conflicts. It is, then, only natural that those conflicts were the ones first taken up by psychoanalysis in Western society. In the words of D. W. Winnicott: 'In psychoanalytic theory ego mechanisms of defence largely belong to the idea of a child that has an independence, a truly personal defence organization.'[8] Psychoanalytic therapy also in its classical form works best when the pathology does not involve dependency; that is, when the patient is potentially independent and only dependent because of his pathology. To quote from Anna Freud: 'Where the phase of dependence has never been overcome and independence has not first been reached and then lost again, it becomes impossible to cure in analysis the state of dependency.'[9] The psychoanalytic situation itself seems to be so structured that one experiences once for all separation from the objects upon which one has depended and thus attains one's own identity. Leo Stone wrote in his recent monograph on the psychoanalytic situation as follows: '. . . the psychoanalytic setting in its general and primary transference impact tends to reproduce, from the outset, the repetitive phases of the state of relative separation from early objects, and most crucially, via the phenomenon of extreme exaggeration, that period of life where all the modalities of bodily intimacy and direct dependence on the mother are being relinquished or attenuated, *pari passu* with the rapid development of the great vehicle of communication by speech'.[10] Thus one may conclude from all the arguments presented heretofore that the Japanese will not warm up to psychoanalytic therapy since they always tend not to accept separation and wish to continue dependency in one form or another. The fact that the Japanese generally tend to trust non-verbal communication more than verbal communication also will make them less available to psychoanalytic therapy.

Truly, such has been the fate of psychoanalysis in Japan until recently. But perhaps there is a change in the air these days. For since the end of the last war many young psychiatrists have been drawn to the study of psychoanalysis. A new series of the translation of Freud's works and many other books on psychoanalysis have been published. Some medical schools have psychoanalytically oriented psychiatrists on their staff. It is also not at all rare nowadays to see patients making request for psychoanalytic therapy. This new entering of psychoanalysis on the Japanese scene has been specifically due to the direct influence of American psychiatry, but more generally it has been facilitated by a rapidly progressing modernization of present-day Japan. Now modernization virtually means Westernization for all non-Western countries and Japan is no exception to this rule. Thus the ideal of 'Western Man' is no longer only Western. This infusion of the Western ideal has been most pronounced in the political area. For the nationalistic fervor which is rallying the people of the non-Western world against the West is inspired by the ideal of independence and freedom, which in itself is really a spiritual heritage of the West. I think the fact that the non-Western countries, as Japan did, often rebel against the West in the name of their sacred tradition does not contradict the above statement. Because the truth is that they believed that they could gain the 'independence' from the West only by reviving their tradition. Again because of the nationalism, the non-Western world is vigorously adopting Western culture on a large scale. I think in Japan this spiritual ferment has shifted from the political sphere to the personal sphere. Thus we see many educated men and women professing such an ideal of independence and freedom for themselves. Such change in the cultural mores of Japan has been responsible for creating the climate favorable to the practice of psychoanalytic therapy.

Should one then congratulate for the sake of psychoanalytic therapy that the favorable conditions for its practice are on the horizon everywhere throughout the world? But a curious thing is that an inverse reaction seems to be taking place in Western society. It is known that the West has experienced a great turmoil and confusion, politically as well as culturally, since the beginning of this century. Thus Western people are no more sure of the permanence, if not the rationale of those values which they have held for centuries. In this predicament, it is interesting, some of them turn to Oriental mysticism, particularly Zen, which promises to abolish the appearance of a solitary and anxiety-ridden selfhood alienated from others and the world. Such people are perhaps numerically rare, but I should think their existence is indicative of a profound change that is shaking up Western society. Speaking, then, of psychoanalytic therapy, we sometimes hear the comment expressed in some professional circles that the orthodox method is too frustrating for most patients. It is feared that psychoanalytic therapy will further alienate them by forcing them to separate from their tenuous object relations. Supportive and anaclitic therapy have come into vogue instead. Of course, one can argue that the recent trend is not a matter of vogue, but is the result of taking more severe cases than ordinary neuroses as the object of psychotherapy. It certainly is. But I wonder if there is something more to this, for even among orthodox analysts there has now emerged a new emphasis on the analyst's helping function, as can be seen, for instance, in Leo Stone's discussion of the parental component in the analyst's identity[11] or Maxwell Gitelson's discussion of the analytic-diatrophic position of the analyst.[12] These new developments, it seems to me, are possibly suggestive of the underlying historical change that the Western ideal of an independent and free person is no more securely shared by all in the West, if much less by patients. This is happening quite ironically at the very time when such an ideal is being adopted, if not in substance at least as a slogan, by the non-Western world.

It is well to remember here, however, that at the time when psychoanalysis was first invented by Freud the cataclysm of the Western world was already under way. One can recall in this regard names like Nietzsche and Kierkegaard. Is not the development of psychoanalysis also related to this cultural and social crisis? Heinz Hartmann, reflecting on the question of why psychoanalysis emerged at the time it did, stated as follows: 'Apparently at certain points in history the ego can no longer cope with its environment, particularly not with that which it itself has created: the means and goal of life lose their orderly relation, and the ego then attempts to fulfil its organizing function by increasing its insight into the inner world.'[13] In other words, psychoanalysis was an attempt of the ego to re-collect itself *vis-à-vis* the demoralizing world. But, one may ask, would it be of any use if the means and goal of life keep losing their orderly relation?

Pertinently, Hartmann continues after the sentence quoted above: 'When is this condition an expression of a collective ego weakness and when is it due to an above-average environmental burden on the ego, are questions which we will by-pass here.' I think one can say that both Nietzsche and Kierkegaard interpreted this condition as symptomatic of a collective ego weakness, the former proclaiming a new morality of superman and the latter a leap unto faith in God in order to strengthen a weak ego. But Freud was on the side of those who took the view that the ego can be strong enough to carry the burden that fell to it in the modern world. Karl Marx can also be said to have held this view. Thus Freud decidedly allied himself with the scientific *Weltanschauung*, putting all his hope for mankind in the progress of science.[14] Psychoanalysis, a science of his creation, should serve this purpose. But this very hope, which was shared by many people of this century, is declining at this moment of history for various reasons. The decline of this hope has then undermined the identity of the psychoanalyst because of his formal alliance with the scientific *Weltanschauung*. I think it is precisely because of this that the psychoanalyst sometimes finds himself in a defensive position in this present-day world. Thus he cannot not only count on the presence of the patient's wish to be independent and free, but he himself can no longer be so sure about the independence of his own position.

How should the psychoanalyst cope with this crisis? I think he cannot excuse himself from facing it by trying to weather the storm in the outside world sitting in his cozy niche. Rather he should admit to himself in all honesty and humility that it was after all his *faith* in reason or the scientific method rather than reason itself that has sustained his independence. He inherited this faith from his predecessors and it worked for quite a while. To begin with, it is clear that Freud had faith in reason and his method when he stated that he had been able to help people with whom he had nothing in common, neither nationality, education, social position nor outlook upon life in general. Naturally, Freud also got his faith from somewhere, but all his followers in psychoanalysis seem to have imbibed his faith. Now suddenly they are awakened to the fact that reason may not stand on its own and might fail them miserably. Will they lose faith in reason? Of course not. They cannot do so without ceasing to be psychoanalysts. But then how can they fix their faith in reason? It seems that even the faith in reason does not come by itself. Or does it? This is a philosophical question which I cannot go into here. At any rate, it can be said that the faith in reason needs to be cared and tended like any other faith. So I think it is a good thing that the psychoanalyst has come to realize that his independence is not inviolable. Because only then he will be able both to cherish his independence truly and to sympathize from his heart with dependent patients. In psychoanalytic therapy, if one should come to the last analysis of what happens there, it is perhaps such a genuine faith in reason on the part of the analyst that is imparted to the patient to make him really independent and free. Freud gave a voice to this idea a long time ago: 'Where id was, there shall ego be.'[15] It was a proclamation of his faith, the faith which represented, as Hartmann pointed out, 'a cultural-historical tendency'.[16]

NOTES

1.   Freud, Sigmund: 'Turnings in the ways of psychoanalytic therapy.' *Collected Papers*, Vol. 2, p. 399. London: The Hogarth Press, 1950.
2.   Doi, L. Takeo: 'Amae – a key concept for understanding Japanese personality structure.' In: *Japanese Culture: Its Development and Characteristics* (Smith, Robert J., and Beardsley, Richard K., eds.). Chicago: Aldine Publishing Co., 1962. See also: 'Japanese language as an expression of Japanese psychology'.*Western Speech*, Spring 1956, 90-96; 'Some thoughts on helplessness and the desire to be loved'. *Psychiatry*, 1963, 26, 266-272.
3.   Freud, Sigmund: *The Future of an Illusion*. A Doubleday Anchor Book.
4.   Freud, Sigmund: *Das Unbehagen in der Kultur*. Fischer Bucherei.
5.   Balint, Michael: 'Critical notes on the theory of the pregenital organizations of the libido'. In: *Primary Love and Psychoanalytic Technique*. New York: Liveright Publishing Corporation, 1953.
6.   Balint, Michael: 'The final goal of psychoanalytic treatment', ibid.
7.   See ref. 5, p. 69.
8.   D. W. Winnicott: 'The theory of the parent-infant relationship'. *Int. J. Psychoanal.*, 1960, 41, 585-595 (at p. 587).
9.   Freud, Anna: 'The theory of the parent-infant relationship – contributions to discussion'. *Int. J. Psychoanal.*, 1962, 43, 240-242 (at p. 242).
10.   Stone, Leo: *The Psychoanalytic Situation*, p. 86. New York: International Universities Press Inc., 1961.
11.   *Ibid.*, p. 44.
12.   Gitelson, Maxwell: 'The first phase of psychoanalysis'. *Int. J. Psychoanal.*, 1962, 43, 194-205.
13.   Hartmann, Heinz: *Ego Psychology and the Problem of Adaptation*, p. 71. New York: International Universities Press Inc., 1958.
14.   Freud, Sigmund: *A Philosophy of Life. New Introductory Lectures on Psychoanalysis*. New York: W. W. Norton & Co., 1933.
15.   *Ibid.*, p. 112.
16.   See ref. 13, p. 71.

First published in R.P. Dore (ed), *Aspects of Social Change*. © Princeton University Press, 1967

⑦ *Giri-Ninjō*: An Interpretation

If one wants to study changes in the nature of interpersonal relations in Japan since 1870, one should ideally compare the material prior to 1870 with the material of succeeding periods up to the present day. My discipline being psychiatry, I have no dearth of contemporary clinical material, but comparable evidence from earlier periods is totally lacking. My alternative is to look at the history of certain concepts which my clinical experience has shown to be crucial, notably *amaeru* and *sumanai*, *giri* and *ninjō*. I propose to show the relation between the first two, expressions of states of mind, to the last two, descriptive of types of interpersonal bonds, an examination of which is essential to the understanding of changes in interpersonal relations since 1870.

AMAERU AND *SUMANAI*

I have described elsewhere[1] the central importance of the concepts of *amaeru* and *sumanai* for the understanding of Japanese patterns of emotion. To summarize the argument briefly:

Amaeru can be translated 'to depend and presume on another's love. . . . . . to seek and bask in another's indulgence'. It is an expression of what the British psychoanalyst Michael Balint calls 'passive object love',[2] a basic ingredient, in his theory, of all psychopathology. Though sometimes translated as 'wheedling', note that the object of this behavior is to receive love itself, not to manipulate a relationship for some other end.

The word is typically used of the behavior of a child toward its mother, but it may also be used of the behavior of lover to lover, of subordinate to master. The word is only rarely used for the behavior of a social superior to a social inferior. The social superior may, however, have an *amaeru* type of emotional dependency on an inferior; in fact he often does. But as a rule he has to guard against revealing it either to himself or to others.

Balint notes that European languages have no word for this passive object love. Japanese has, and the availability of the word makes it easy for Japanese patients to express the wish to be loved and to become aware of it, and also for the therapist to detect that wish. By contrast, according to Balint, although Western patients may have the same passive desire to be loved they come to accept and gratify it only after a lengthy painstaking analysis.

The linguistic difference does reflect a difference in social relations. In Japan the dependency of children on parents is fostered even beyond the nursing period and institutionalized. It is not the case, however, that the desire to be loved is always gratified. The variety of phrases to describe distortions or frustrations of that desire is evidence enough.[3] They do, however, serve to reinforce the impression that the Japanese are preoccupied with this desire.

Sumanai, more politely *sumimasen*, caught the attention of Ruth Benedict[4] because it is used on occasions when English speakers would use three different expressions: 'I feel guilty', 'I am sorry', and 'thank you'. Apart from its use as an expletive, the same word, as the negative form of the verb *sumu*, may be used to say that a debt is 'not paid off' or that a task 'is uncompleted'.

Benedict, noting these other uses of the word and the parallel they implicitly draw between financial and moral debts, explained the use of this word to mean 'thank you' by saying that it expressed one's sense of indebtedness accompanied by a painful realization that repayment is required some day.

She may be right that there is this ambivalence, but my analysis of Japanese neurotic patients has led me to suspect an ambivalence of a different kind related to the feelings expressed in *amaeru* behavior. If one has caused another person real harm or trouble, then the expression *sumanai*, standing for 'I am sorry' or 'I feel guilty', is a natural expression of a sense that one has not done as one ought to have done. But I have observed neurotic patients to use the word in this sense when the harm or trouble they have caused is imaginary. In these cases they secretly harbor hostile feelings toward the other which have been caused by frustration of their wish to *amaeru*. To say *sumanai* wards off such feelings; it implores the other not to drop one from grace despite one's fault (i.e., one's hostility). As such it is a disguised expression of the desire to *amaeru*. Likewise, *sumanai* where an English speaker would say 'thank you' is an acknowledgment that one has indeed caused the other trouble inasmuch as the favor received is at his expense, and simultaneously a request that the other should not drop one from grace in spite of his loss.

NINJŌ AND *GIRI*

When Benedict spoke of the concept of 'human feelings' in Japanese culture and included in it all the natural impulses and inclinations of man, she was presumably referring to the word *ninjō*, which etymologically means 'human feelings'. But *ninjō* to the Japanese means a much more specific constellation of feeling and one which is looked on by Japanese specifically as Japanese. (Hence comments to the effect that Westerners 'do not understand' or 'also have' *ninjō*.) In my interpretation *ninjō* means specifically knowing how to *amaeru* properly and how to respond to the call of *amaeru* in others. Japanese think themselves especially sensitive to these feelings, and those who do not share that sensitivity are said to be wanting in *ninjō*.

Giri, by contrast, refers to a bond of moral obligation (whether or not of a kind specific to Japanese society is a controversy which need not concern us here). Thus, whereas *ninjō* primarily refers to those feelings which spontaneously occur in the relations between parent and child, husband and wife, or brothers and sisters, *giri* relations are relations between in-laws, neighbors, with close associates, or superiors in one's place of work. However, there is an inner connection between the two. Family relations also have an aspect to which the term *giri* can be applied, and at the same time *ninjō* can be extended to *giri* relations. In other words *giri* relations are pseudo-*ninjō* relations in which one may – and ideally always seeks to – experience *ninjō*. One may never, or only seldom, succeed, and usually one is left only with the semblance of *ninjō* and frustration of one's desire to *amaeru*, yet nevertheless the ideal is worth striving for. Interestingly enough, it is in *giri* relations that one would experience the feelings expressed as *sumanai* very frequently. This, I think, nicely illustrates the point that has been made above, that is: *giri* relations are pseudo-*ninjō* relations, since *sumanai* indicates the frustrated desire to *amaeru* seeking to express itself.

In this connection I would like to point out a few misleading remarks made by Benedict and shared by others; for instance, the notion that 'the circle of human feelings' and 'the circle of duty' are mutually exclusive. At times they may appear to be mutually exclusive, but *giri* relations are really there in order to be pervaded by *ninjō*. In this regard, Dore's assertion[5] that, for the male, the family belonged to the circle of 'duty', and male friendships to the circle of 'human feelings', also obscures the psychological interrelations of *giri* and *ninjō* by making the same assumption of mutual exclusiveness. What is more, I think that if one were to ask a modern Japanese to label family life and male friendships according to *giri* and *ninjō*, he would rather reverse Dore's classification. This again does not mean that the family never freezes into mere *giri* relations devoid of *ninjō* or that male friendships never flourish into *ninjō*. Such possibilities clearly suggest that the circle of *giri* and that of *ninjō* are not fixed, but fluid; also that these two concepts refer to states of affairs rather than to kinds of personal relations. Finally, Benedict's statement[6] that 'these old tales of times when *giri* was from the heart and had no taint of resentment are modern Japan's daydream of a golden age' is quite misleading. It is true that many *giri* relations are just a semblance of what they are supposed to be, but this fact does not prevent some *giri* relations from being entirely satisfactory to each partner because they are suffused with *ninjō*. It is such satisfactory *giri* relations which the Japanese usually understand by the term of friendship.

HISTORICAL CHANGES AND THE TRADITIONAL PATTERNS OF BEHAVIOR

Modern Japan underwent two critical transformations, the Meiji Restoration and the defeat in The Second World War, which had immense effects on traditional patterns of interpersonal relations. At the time of the Meiji Restoration the emperor system or *kokutai* was formally established and came to constrain the traditional patterns of behavior – those centered upon *giri* and *ninjō*. Because the emperor was now a deity,[7] dedication and loyalty to him (loyalty was originally a feature of personal *giri* relations) became an absolute duty (*gimu*) that should take precedence over *giri* and *ninjō* in ordinary human relations. This emperor system, I think, served a double function in terms of individuation in modern Japan. On the one hand, it apparently promoted the individuation of the Japanese, inasmuch as it gave a rallying point for every individual, irrespective of social status, family, sex, or education. But on the other hand, and this was more important, it hindered individuation since it subjected every individual to the emperor by a spiritual bond and did not allow him to establish his independent self apart from this bond.

Now thanks to the defeat in the last war, the emperor system has been abolished. Being freed from the mysterious bond that tied them to the emperor, people also began to question the validity of all traditional morals, especially the morals of *giri* and *ninjō*. With this questioning, however, it seems that people have become even more acutely aware of the frustration of their desires to *amaeru*, since previously their personal conflicts were supposed to be absorbed into personal dedication and loyalty to the emperor. The following example is particularly interesting in this regard. One of my patients said that he would like to have somebody who would take the responsibility of doing *hohitsu* with him. *Hohitsu* is a special legal term which was used for the act of assisting the emperor with his task of governing the nation, and in this task his subordinates took all the responsibility, leaving none to the emperor. In other words, the emperor's position, psychologically speaking, signified the absolute gratification of dependency wishes. Of course, prior to the abolition of the emperor system, nobody thought that way or envied the emperor for that matter. But now the emperor being no deity, my patient intuitively sensed the psychological meaning of the emperor's position and used the word *hohitsu* to reveal his deep frustration of the desire to *amaeru*.

Removing the strait jacket of *kokutai* had definitely made people more vulnerable to internal conflicts. Also, without the support of *kokutai* for one's identity, the onslaught of various ideologies in Western civilization has to be faced individually. Thus we have in modern Japan the chaotic influx of various 'isms' and faiths superimposed on the intricate entanglements of *giri* and *ninjō*. There is, for instance, increased self-assertion or pursuit of self-interest emerging out of the conflicts over *giri* and *ninjō*. This new trend is usually associated in the minds of the Japanese with individualism, one of the Western ideologies imported into Japan. It seems to me, however, that this trend amounts in most cases to what I would describe as an extreme pursuit of the desire to *amaeru*, accompanied by another emotion, that of suspicion and mistrust toward others. I do not mean to say in this regard that such individualism is only a peculiarly Japanese phenomenon and does not exist in the West. I also cannot discuss here how it compares with the original spirit of individualism as it developed in the West. At any rate, the post-war trend has made one crucial conflict manifest, that is, the conflict over *amaeru* or that of whether one is loved or not. I say this conflict is crucial because one's self-respect in the final analysis hinges upon its successful solution. Only when one is certain on this score is one able to stand as an independent individual.

In this connection it is interesting to recall a recent comment by Masao Maruyama that almost all Japanese leaders in all walks of life are convinced that they are always surrounded by hostile critics, a consciousness which Maruyama calls 'an ever-present sense of being wronged by others' (*higaisha ishiki*).[8] This fact clearly indicates that all of these people harbor the desire to *amaeru* and feel frustrated in it. If the leading representatives of Japanese society are like this, how would the rest feel, not to speak of those patients who come to seek help from psychiatrists? Perhaps if there was anything defective in the working of the traditional patterns of behavior centered in *giri* and *ninjō*, it was the fact that it did not solve the conflict over whether one is loved or not, rather perpetuated it, since *giri* by its nature binds people in dependent relationships and *ninjō* only encourages dependency. The fact, then, that the Japanese are blessed with such a word as *amaeru* may not be a measure of their satisfaction after all, but rather of their preoccupation with it because of dissatisfaction. But then the question remains: how does one solve the conflict over one's dependency wishes? Would it be by acquiring the inner certainty of being loved once for all or by dispensing with dependency wishes altogether? I cannot discuss this matter any further, since it touches upon a more philosophical question of how individualism developed in the West in the first place and of what is the nature of individuation. At any rate, if Japanese society should proceed toward more individuation, I should think that it will not be simply by dint of industrialization, but by searching deeply into the foundations of Western culture.

NOTES

1. See L T. Doi, '*Amae*: A Key Concept for Understanding Japanese Personality Structure', in Smith and Beardsley, *Japanese Culture* (Chicago, 1962).
2. M. Balint, *Primary Love and Psychoanalytic Technique* (London, 1952), p. 69.
3. See the analysis of *suneru, higamu, hinekureru, tereru, toriiru, tanoma, kodawaru*, and *amanzuru* in Doi, '*Amae*'.
4. Ruth Benedict, *The Chrysanthemum and the Sword* (Boston, 1946).
5. *City Life in Japan* (London, 1958), pp. 175-76.

6.   Ruth Benedict, *The Chrysanthemum and the Sword*, p. 139.

7.   I believe that the national myth of the emperor as 'God' was really created at the time of the Meiji Restoration, even though it appeared on the surface that this was only an official restatement of a Japanese myth about the emperor's being *kami*. In other words, I would like to stress the point that the form of emperor worship we held after the Meiji Restoration would possibly never have been established were it not for the impact of Western civilization upon Japan. It is well known that Western civilization became the model for Japan to copy from, whether this civilization was introduced in the form of science, technical skills, religion, individualism, democracy, or communism. The establishment of the emperor system was a special case in the Westernization of Japan. In fact, there is good historical evidence that the nature of the authority which Meiji statesmen invested in the emperor was really borrowed from their image of Western civilization, especially Christianity, in order to cope with it. (See Maruyama, Masao, *Nihon no shisō*, 1961, pp. 28-31.) At any rate, at the Privy Council in 1889, when the draft of the first constitution of Japan was introduced, Prince Ito had this to say: neither Buddhism nor Shintoism could play the role which Christianity was playing in Western countries as the basis for their constitutional governments. He then proposed that in Japan only the emperor could serve as the basis of the constitution, thus fulfilling the role of religion in Western countries. It was for this reason, I believe, that the emperor was officially held as sacred by the first constitution.

8.   *Nihon no shisō*, pp. 14-44.

First published in W. Caudill and Tsung-yi Lin (eds), *Mental Health Research in Asia and the Pacific*, Honolulu, East-West Center, 1969

⑧ Japanese Psychology, Dependency Need and Mental Health

In previous papers I have stressed dependency need as a keynote of the Japanese personality structure (Doi, 1962, 1963, 1964). I arrived at this conclusion from analysis of Japanese patients, using the concept of *amaeru*, a common Japanese verb which usually describes what a small child feels toward his parents and also the similar feeling that may exist between two adults. The uniqueness of this concept and its usage seem to suggest that dependency need is quite accessible and acceptable to the consciousness of the average Japanese person. To put it the other way round, there seems to be a social sanction for dependency need in Japanese society. If this is the case for Japanese society, it clearly contrasts with the situation in Western societies where dependency need is looked upon as something that belongs to the child or the regressed patient and, hence, usually beneath the dignity of a grown-up person.

It is interesting that relatively few textbooks on child psychology written in Western countries refer to dependency need as such. They treat the emotional development of children at great length, but the dependency need which seems to the Japanese so elemental and basic for children is not given sufficient attention. In spite of a recent emphasis placed upon the mother-child relation and the importance of the child's emotional tie to the mother, the dependency need that should underlie such a bond is seldom mentioned. It may be true to the picture of such a cultural climate to state that it is as though a conspiracy eager to banish dependency need from the adult world had almost succeeded in eliminating it even from the child world.

Turning to psychoanalytic literature, however, it is apparent that in it the dependence of children upon their parents is duly recognized. Freud wrote in 1926: 'The biological factor is the long period of time during which the young of the human species is in a condition of helplessness and dependency. . . . This biological factor, then, establishes the earliest situation of danger and creates the need to be loved which will accompany the child through the rest of its life.' This need to be loved which Freud mentioned certainly seems to be the same as dependency need. It is interesting to recall, however, that dependence, as such, did not at first

53

suggest the presence of a dependency need to Freud, for in 1915 he wrote that the primal narcissistic condition would not have come into being 'were it not that every individual goes through a period of helplessness and dependence on fostering care, during which his urgent needs are satisfied by agencies outside himself and thereby withheld from developing along their own line'. According to Freud, it is as though one could depend on fostering care without having a need on one's part for such a dependency; only secondarily would one develop the need to be loved because of the danger inherent in the state of dependency. Hence, in his thinking both loving and being loved came to be defined in terms of libidinal satisfaction (Freud, 1914, 1915).

Against this theory of Freud's, I propose that dependency need should be thought of as an independent drive, distinct from the sexual or aggressive drives, from which develops the need to be loved. In psychoanalytic terminology the sexual and aggressive drives usually are referred to as id impulses, whereas I believe that dependency need should be thought as deriving from ego; that is, it corresponds to the ego instincts in Freud's early formulation. I cannot help feeling that Freud discarded the concept of the ego instincts later, mainly because he could not appreciate the independent importance of dependency need. Now, though conceptually separated, sexual and aggressive drives, on the one hand, and dependency need, on the other, work together and are intertwined with each other in actuality. It can be presumed that object relations, which sexual and aggressive drives require for proper satisfaction, come into being by means of the operation of dependency need. It follows, then, that the pathology of dependency need comes first in individual psychopathology, and that either sex or aggression is secondary. This reasoning agrees with recent studies of animal behavior in which animals deprived of mothers from birth cannot develop proper sexual activities (Harlow and Harlow, 1962). Pathology must reside in ego first and foremost, whether in psychosis or neurosis, though id impulses greatly contribute to it. I feel also that such Freudian concepts as narcissism, homosexuality, masochism, unconscious guilt, and repetition compulsion, concepts which, though ill defined, are important for understanding the dynamics of psychopathology, need to be revised in terms of dependency need (Doi, 1965).

I have attempted to do with the concept of dependency need what Freud did with that of sexuality. He made it possible to conceive the whole development in continuum from infancy to adulthood in terms of sexuality, or more technically libido, by giving that concept adequate abstraction and generality. This procedure is what gives psychoanalysis the status of science, for, as Langer (1964) said, 'The sciences are born under quite special conditions when their key concepts reach a degree of abstraction and precision which makes them adequate to the demands of exact, powerful, and microscopically analytic thinking.' I think that this procedure can be applied to the concept of dependency need. I have no doubt been helped in so thinking by the fact that the Japanese language has many words like *amaeru* which express dependency need in its multifarious shades. Without such a cultural background perhaps even Freud, for all his genius, could not easily recognize the importance of dependency need. In his later years, however, he made the following statement (Freud, 1931) concerning his new insight into early mental development: 'Everything connected with this first mother-attachment has in analysis seemed to me so elusive, lost in a past so dim and shadowy, so hard to resuscitate, that it seemed as if it had undergone some specially inexorable repression.' This sentence is a good example of the great difficulty one would experience in identifying dependency need as such in Western societies, though it cannot be determined whether the repression of the dependency need is real or only apparent owing to the observer's lack of acumen, as Freud partially admits in the passage.

I have stated that dependency need should be thought of as an independent drive which makes object relations possible in the first years of life. It follows that the operation of dependency need initiates not only the process of personality formation but also the process of socialization. Heretofore, these two processes could not be integrated theoretically; hence, one was hard put to account for social and cultural factors in personality formation. For instance, Hartmann (1944) commented on this subject:

> Considering this complete dependence upon the care and protection of others, it is natural that man's need for love and his fear of losing the love of the object are especially strongly developed. It is evident that analytic findings of this kind are of great importance for sociology. At the same time when viewed from the angle of adaptation, maturation, and learning, they present an essential field in the biology of man. The relationship of the infant to his mother, the institution of the reality principle, the change in the types of instinctual gratification, may all be described 'biologically' as well as 'sociologically'.

Here, though Hartmann rightly has recognized the phenomena of dependence as a common area of study for sociology and biology, he has provided no working concept to mediate between the two disciplines. Faithfully following Freud, he has not regarded infantile dependency as involving a psychological need that through its own dynamism should promote the process of socialization. No wonder that he mentioned only sociology and biology, not psychology, an omission which probably betrays his hidden assumption that the phenomena of dependence cannot be studied psychologically. Thus in discussing how man can be affected by cultural factors, he simply said: 'They can, along with other influences, co-determine the central structure of the personality, by provoking, for example, the early establishment of specific reaction formations, or they can co-determine the degree of severity of the superego or the decree of mobility of the ego.'

To be precise, one may argue, cultural factors cannot touch the central structure of the personality unless there is some need in the core of the personality which is responsive to and affected by cultural factors. This need is what I mean by dependency need, the need which first involves one's parents but through and beyond them extends to the wider world. I think Balint (1935), whose view is quite similar to mine, had the same thing in mind when he posited passive object love as a primary need and said: 'Now I believe . . . that the different object relations do not succeed one another according to biological conditions, but are to be conceived as reactions to actual influence of the world of objects – above all, to methods of upbringing. Our therapy is the best proof of this.' Thus, through the mediating concept of dependency need it becomes possible to relate social systems and personality systems, and I think this association will open a new vista for cultural anthropology and also for mental health.

In the light of the above hypothesis, let us consider some of the culturally conditioned personality types. I contrasted at the beginning of this chapter the attitudes of Japanese society and Western societies toward dependency need. I also suggested the possible existence of a certain bias against dependency need in Western societies – a bias which must be related to the Western ideal of personal independence. I cannot give here a detailed historical account of the reasons such an ideal came to exist in Western societies. Perhaps it has to do with the fact that the West has gone through more turbulent social and cultural changes throughout its history than has the East, thus creating a suitable climate for the spirit of personal independence. To state this spirit in dynamic terms, it means that one might just as well depend upon oneself or become independent, since there is nobody else to depend upon. In other words, personal independence is the dependency need turned upon oneself, and its viability as a defense presupposes the existence of a self worthy to be depended upon; this latter point is a crucial one for psychopathology. Furthermore, I think that the spirit of personal independence has been the driving force behind all the great cultural achievements of the West, rather than 'the increase in autonomy of the ego' or freedom from instinctual conflicts which Hartmann, Kris, and Loewenstein (1951) have associated with the ability for higher mental functions. If anything, personal independence creates even more mental conflicts than does dependence, though it may subsequently check them successfully or unsuccessfully.

I now return to the discussion of the problem with which I started, that is, the ego-syntonic quality of dependency need in the Japanese personality structure, particularly with reference to remarks made by other Asiatics in this volume. For instance, Surya (Chapter 23) stresses the importance of dependent relations for Indians, but he cautions against the use of the word 'dependency', because it has a bad connotation. According to him, the right words are bond, bondship, or kinship rather than dependency, and an Indian would not experience dependency but anticipation of closeness or bondship in the act of asking for a favor. This reasoning implies, it seems to me, that Indians share the same bias toward dependency need as do Westerners. Also, if Surya's interpretation is correct, what he describes as characteristic of Indians is intensive identification with one's group, and I am sure that the same group identification characterizes in good measure the Japanese as well. I feel, however, that, eager as the Japanese are to identify themselves with a group to which they belong, they also tend to think in terms of personal interests and often look upon allegiance to a particular group as a burden. They may even try to manipulate their group or others upon whom they depend, so as to turn their dependency into virtual control of others. In other words, the Japanese dependent relations are quite fluid, and the structure of these relations does not necessarily consist of the fixed social roles of a dependent and a superior. A person in a superior role may as easily experience dependency need as a person in a dependent role as part of the interaction. This structure is as it should be in terms of dependency need, for one establishes a close bond or a group identification more often than not at the expense of one's individual wishes, and I am inclined to believe that this structure is what distinguishes the Japanese pattern of dependency from those found in the rest of Asia.

The fact that the Japanese people have eagerly and readily welcomed Western civilization since the Meiji period is an indication of the value they place on the free play of initiative. I think it would be wrong, however, to infer that Japanese initiative is the same in nature as the Western idea of personal independence. Rather, I should say that their initiative has more to do with dependency than with the need to become independent, since it has been mainly motivated by the desire to appear acceptable and respectable in the eyes of others. In other words, the Japanese have accomplished the task of modernizing themselves by use of the surplus free energy of dependency need which is neither bound by any specific social relation nor turned upon oneself to make self-reliance workable. To prove this point, let us briefly examine the case of the recent war Japan waged against her neighbors. Without exhausting the list of the causes that entered into making this war, one could say that Japan wanted to be recognized as one of the world powers. Short of such recognition, she wanted to act as though she were a world power. In her eyes therefore the course of action she eventually took was an act of identification with the aggressor. Take also the case of the remarkable transformation which has come over the face of Tokyo during the past few years. It is no secret to the citizens of Tokyo that the change was made possible by the tremendous incentive that came from the honor of having the Olympic games there. Japan has always been like that. In fact, she made similar successful efforts in the past when she was confronted with a great civilization in China. From the Japanese example one may therefore hazard the thesis that a key to successful modernization of any country less developed than others lies in the inherent strength or relative health of dependency among its people.

At present the whole non-Western world is straining under the impact of

Western civilization. While this social cataclysm goes on in the non-Western world, the West also is passing through a critical phase. For one thing, the West can no longer *depend* upon its cherished hegemony of the world. To maintain this hegemony, it preaches to or sells to or even forces upon the rest of the world the ideal of democracy, or whatever it may be, only to find more confusion created. It is little wonder, then, that at times the ideal sounds hollow even to the West itself. Thus the whole world rapidly is becoming one in political, social, and cultural confusion, for which the West has to take at least part of the blame. This situation also means, however, that conditions are hopefully again ripe for a rediscovery of the spirit of personal independence, the source of so much creativity in the West. I think that is why the people in Western societies are so eagerly seeking new meanings of emotional maturity and have to flock to psychoanalysts or to whatever promises them a complete self-realization.

As for the Japanese people, they also are not really content with their accomplishment of modernization. Since they have embraced Western civilization with all its dilemmas and conflicts, they are learning, almost despite themselves, the hard lessons that they cannot completely depend upon others whom they once looked upon as superior and that they have to acquire spiritual independence somewhere or somehow in order to cope with the cultural and social confusion. I think that the social instability now being experienced in Japan goes hand in hand with a recent increase in psychiatric casualties. What can be done to meet this emerging situation? Of course, all the facilities in the field of mental health will have to be mobilized and expanded, for it is the task of mental health workers to help those who stumble and fall by the wayside in this historical process of mankind. But how? With what philosophy? Or with what technology? Are we psychiatrists well equipped for the job? Does our work consist mainly in building more hospitals or producing an abundance of tranquilizers? I think the answer to this critical question which confronts us all today is obvious. It must be first and foremost to educate an increasing number of psychiatrists and other workers in the field of mental health toward a better understanding of the human mind, particularly to help them overcome their own sometimes unrecognized dependency need. Such education is essential because only those who are truly conflict-free in respect to dependency need, and therefore able to make use of it in creative ways, are able to understand and help others who suffer from the frustration of dependency need.

REFERENCES

Balint, M. 1935. Critical notes on the theory of the pregenital organizations of the libido. Reprinted in *Primary love and psychoanalytic technique*. M. Balint. New York, Liveright Publishing Company, 1965.
Doi, L.T. 1962. *Amae* – a key concept for understanding Japanese personality structure. In

Japanese culture: its development and characteristics. R.J. Smith and R. K. Beardsley, eds. Chicago, Aldine Publishing Company.

—— 1963. Some thoughts on helplessness and the desire to be loved. *Psychiatry* 26:266-72.

—— 1964. *Psychoanalytic therapy and 'Western Man': a Japanese view.* Special Edition No. 1 (Congress Issue) of the *International Journal of Social Psychiatry.* Pp. 13-18.

—— 1965. *Seishin-bunseki to seishin-byōro.* Tokyo, Igaku Shoin.

Freud, S. 1914. On narcissism: an introduction. Reprinted in *Collected papers.* Vol. 4. London, The Hogarth Press, 1950.

—— 1915. Instincts and their vicissitudes. Reprinted in *Collected papers.* Vol. 4. London, The Hogarth Press, 1950.

—— 1926. *Inhibitions, symptoms and anxiety.* London, the Hogarth Press.

—— 1931. Female sexuality. Reprinted in *Collected papers.* Vol. 5. London, The Hogarth Press, 1950.

Harlow, H. F., and M. K. Harlow. 1962. The effect of rearing conditions on behavior. *Bulletin of the Menninger Clinic* 26:213-24.

Hartmann, H. 1944. Psychoanalysis and sociology. Reprinted in *Essays on ego psychology.* H. Hartmann. New York, International Universities Press. 1964.

Hartmann, H., E. Kris, and R. M. Loewenstein. 1951. Some psychoanalytic comments on culture and personality. In *Psychoanalysis and culture.* G. B. Wilbur and W. Muensterberger, eds. New York, International Universities Press.

Langer, S. K. 1964. *Philosophical sketches,* p. 13. New York, Mentor Books.

—— 1965. Introduction to mental hygiene. Quezon City, Phoenix Publishing House.

Wittkower E. D., and J. Fried. 1959. A cross-cultural approach to mental health problems. *American Journal of Psychiatry* 116:423-28.

Yap, P. M. 1952. The latah reaction: its pathodynamics and nosological position. *Journal of Mental Science* 98:515-64.

Zarco, R. M. 1959. A sociological study of illegal narcotic activity in the Philippines. Unpublished M.S. thesis, University of the Philippines.

Zigler, E., and L. Phillips. 1961a. Psychiatric diagnosis and symptomatology. *Journal of Abnormal and Social Psychology* 63:69 75.

—— 1961b. Psychiatric diagnosis: a critique. *Journal of Abnormal and Social Psychology* 63:607-18.

First published in *Solidarity,* Vol.6, No.8, August 1971

⑨ A Psychiatrist's View on *Zeitgeist*

I t is true that the present sophistication of psychiatry makes us believe that the troubled people and the troubled world are not things apart but very closely related. So much so that we feel we cannot fully understand the troubled people without taking account of the troubled world. It was not, however, always like that. In previous times the function of a psychiatrist was confined to the care of the mentally sick, segregated in remote hospitals from society at large, who could be nicely classified as schizophrenics, manic-depressives, obsessives, hysterics, hypochondriacs, etc. Nowadays the mentally sick are everywhere, in and out of hospitals. This means that they have increased in number. Also, many of them do not fit classified categories, an indication that mental illness changes in form, keeping pace with historical and social changes. Interestingly, even those who fit into classified categories sometimes can manage to live their 'normal' lives, thanks to the improvement of treatment methods. What is ironical is the fact that in this rapidly changing age one can no longer take for granted what is normal. No wonder then that the boundary between the normal and the abnormal is blurred if not altogether extinct.

All these trends, it seems, have contributed to a recent emphasis on social pathology rather than individual psychopathology. What matters is not whether an individual becomes sick or not, but whether the whole society is healthy for individual members or not. Since our society naturally has many shortcomings in this respect, the notion of a sick society was born and it has become very popular among educated people. For this reason, the American Psychiatric Association invited Stuart Hughes, a distinguished Harvard professor of history, to their annual meeting last year and heard his lecture on 'Emotional Disturbance and American Change, 1944-69'. To contradict what the audience might have expected to hear, Prof. Hughes sharply criticized the popular notion of a sick society, saying that 'it is vague to the point of meaninglessness', that 'it provides no guidelines for the future', that 'it suggests a despair of reason itself'. He then poses the following question: 'If we are sick people living in a sick society, then we need physicians, and psychiatrists are the only doctors available. But if the complaint is as general and unspecific as fashionable rhetoric suggests, how are the psychiatrists to diagnose and treat it? How can they possibly minister to a whole population?'

Prof. Hughes is justified in detecting irresponsibility in the notion of a sick society and also in chiding psychiatrists gently for their possible presumption for not doing anything about it. But by thus criticizing the contemporary notion of a sick society, isn't Prof. Hughes making his own diagnosis of the present society? In other words, one can say just as well, according to Prof. Hughes' verdict, that the contemporary people are 'sick' precisely because they are content with calling their own society sick. His diagnosis on our society is more accurate than what is usually given by psychiatrists. However, this 'sickness' is not beyond psychiatric comprehension, notwithstanding Prof. Hughes' statement. As a matter of fact it can be conceptualized in psychiatric terms, though it may not be cured by ordinary psychiatric treatments.

A particular contemporary sickness would be youth unrest, a world-wide phenomenon which incites many countries, aggravating at times to the point of a civil war. In Japan, for instance, we have had university riots which spread to almost all universities and colleges for the past couple of years. Similar trouble can be found in other countries. Prof. Hughes touches upon this problem of university riots, too, in his above-mentioned lecture and states: 'What has been unusual about the insurgent mood of the past half decade has been its juxtaposition of anarchism and the peremptory silencing of opponents, its peculiar blend of political puritanism and personal licence, its cult of 'confrontation' as a quasi-religious act of witness. Together this complex of attitudes suggests something quite different from the conventional revolutionary aim of seizing the means of production or the implements of power and redirecting them for the benefit of the masses. It suggests, rather, a basically unpolitical aspiration to see through, to unmask, to strip – literally as well as figuratively – down to total nakedness. The goal is psychological or, to use old-fashioned vocabulary, spiritual. And it marks the culmination of a quarter-century of amateur psychologizing among the young.'

This is certainly a very apt description of contemporary youth movement, but Prof. Hughes merely calls it psychological or spiritual, not specifying what kind of psychological or spiritual problem it is. One would like to know, for instance, what really motivates those youths to engage in such activities. In my opinion, they seem to provoke guilt feelings in adults who hold responsible positions by reminding them of their injustices and negligences. For this purpose they try any method and even resort to violence. In fact, violent action is deliberately used as the most effective weapon to provoke guilt feelings in the opponents, because it hurts them, thus making them aware, sometimes for the first time, of their hidden egoism. Those youths who engage in violent action do not feel guilty themselves, because they completely identify themselves with the oppressed, the exploited, the alienated, the under-privileged, the discriminated or the poor depending on the circumstances. In other words, they identify themselves as the victims, too.

61

Does this psychology sound familiar or strange? This is quite familiar to the Japanese. However, they have a special word for it, *higaisha-ishiki*, meaning the consciousness of one who was wronged. *Higaisha*, meaning one who was wronged and its counterpart, *kagaisha*, meaning one who inflicts a wrong on others, are everyday Japanese words and are used more frequently and freely than corresponding English words, the injured party and the perpetrator. The word *higaisha-ishiki* is very popular. This would indicate that the Japanese tend to feel wronged and to dwell on their being imposed upon to the extent that such a state of mind becomes often an important ingredient of their identity. Perhaps the secret of why Japan waged her last war against such a formidable nation like the United States also lies in this psychology. She did so, not because she calculated she could win a war, but only because she wanted her opponent to be involved into war, so that her opponent would feel guilty afterward. One would think that Japan was rather successful in this hidden design, though she suffered terribly because of the war.

The relation between the psychology of youth unrest and the psychology of the Japanese people is not just accidental. What motivates youth now on a world-wide scale in their apparently futile political activities is very much similar to what motivated Japan in her last war; that is, *higaisha-ishiki*. The fact that youth riots have been particularly rampant in Japan proves this point. Even *zengakuren* has inspired youth movements in other countries. The fact then that even the youth in a powerful nation like the United States can indulge in essentially abject feelings of *higaisha-ishiki* can be attributed to several factors: 1) Contemporary youth can no longer identify themselves with their nation, whether powerful or not. 2) Liberation of former colonies gives ample opportunities for youth to identify themselves with the under-privileged and the exploited. 3) Threat of nuclear holocaust makes everybody both defensive and defenseless. 4) Pollution and destruction of nature due to the advance of industrialization and the political use of mass communication make everybody vulnerable. I think these factors have added up to establish the negative identity of *higaisha-ishiki* in youth throughout the world.

The characteristic spirit of the present age is none other than *higaisha-ishiki*. This would appear to be almost insane to those who don't share this feeling. Actually, one might say just as well that it is what paranoiacs feel inside. But to call a paranoiac as such does not cure him. It takes a long and painstaking treatment to cure him and even this does not always succeed. If treating a single patient is difficult, how much more for a whole population caught in *higaisha-ishiki*? Prof. Hughes is right. Psychiatrists can't do a thing about it. But then who will help ill-guided *Zeitgeist*? Let time flow so that it also will flow away?

The polarization of mankind between *higaisha* and *kagaisha* is an artificial yet dangerous one. Furthermore guilt feelings which *higaisha* sometimes succeeds to provoke in *kagaisha* are not dependable. In other words, they do not sink in and will soon evaporate when *kagaisha* turns into *higaisha*, as it is likely to happen. But what if the whole of mankind acquires *higaisha-ishiki*? This could be a logical outcome of contemporary youth movement.

First published in *Psychiatry: Journal for the Study of Interpersonal Processes.* Vol. 35, No. 4, November 1972 © William Alanson White Psychiatric Foundation, Inc.

⑩ A Japanese Interpretation of Erich Segal's *Love Story*[*]

I would like to mention first why I chose to discuss *Love Story*. It is not because I love the story. I cannot even say that it is a great story, worthy of a psychiatrist's serious comment. Certainly it is a popular novel in the United States, and it has become popular in Japan, too, through the movie made from it. In fact, sweet and sad melodramas about heroines used to be common in Japanese films, particularly in prewar days. I think the Japanese audiences have been a bit surprised to find their old familiar theme depicted in a modern American film.

My attention was called to this story in the following manner. The Japanese Council for the Promotion of the Sciences set up a joint research committee of Japanese and American scholars in 1971, the purpose of which was to make a comparative study of the Japanese way of communication and the American way. Soon after, I was asked to join the committee and was told that their current task was to study Erich Segal's *Love Story*, as the Japanese translation was becoming popular with Japanese young people. Subsequently I read the story, saw the movie, and pondered about it. What follows then is my cross-cultural speculation on the story.

Before I go on to the main discussion, I would like to introduce the concept of *amae*, which I shall use extensively in analysis of this story. As explained in my previous publications (1962, 1963, 1964), it means a particular dependency need which manifests itself in a longing to merge with others in a loving relationship. The key word in this definition is *merge*, and it primarily refers to what a child feels or does toward his parents, particularly his mother. But it can also be used to describe the relationship between two adults, such as lovers or a husband and a wife or a master and a pupil. Since it is a uniquely Japanese word, it applies best to descriptions of Japanese interpersonal relationships. But the concept itself is general enough and I think there is no reason why it can't be used to explain the psychology of non-Japanese too. That is exactly what I am attempting to do in this study.

[*] Based on a speech given at the National Institute of Mental Health, Bethesda, Maryland, August 20, 1971.

Love Story is about two young persons, Oliver Barrett IV, the son of a wealthy, well-known banker, and Jenny Cavilleri, the only daughter of an Italian-American widower. They fall in love and soon get married, contrary to the wishes of Oliver's family. It is not that Oliver's family absolutely objects to Oliver's getting married to Jenny; rather, they want Oliver to wait until graduation so that the relationship can stand the test of time. But he will have none of this and from that moment on cuts all his relationships with his family. Now this distresses Jenny no end, who herself is very close to her own father. Or it would be better to say that Jenny and her father simply cannot understand the kind of relationship Oliver has with his father. Oliver in turn cannot understand why they cannot understand him. He says:

> And there I got my first inkling of a cultural gap between us. I mean, three and a half years of Harvard-Radcliff had pretty much made us into the cocky intellectuals that institution traditionally produces, but when it came to accepting the fact that my father was made of stone, she adhered to some atavistic Italian-Mediterranean notion of papa-loves-bambinos, and there was no arguing otherwise.

So, interestingly, this story itself evolves from a kind of cross-cultural problem existing within the United States.

I think the intensity of the fierce competitiveness which Oliver feels toward his father is also beyond comprehension for Japanese. They would even say that the father is not the kind of person who deserves such a reaction from his son. Though called Old Stonyface by Oliver, he is portrayed, as far as the story goes, as a basically kind and understanding person. Then why this outburst of fierce competitiveness? Why this almost violent rivalry on the part of the son toward the father? One might describe it as a typical Oedipal situation, which is technically correct. But to call it Oedipal does not explain the fact that this kind of father-son relationship may be characteristic especially of those who are called W-A-S-P, and not of the Italian-Mediterranean type, nor perhaps of Jewish people, and certainly not of Japanese. I hasten to add, to avoid misunderstanding, that the Japanese father-son relationship is not always smooth and harmonious. Even minus competition, you can still have friction. We have a saying in Japan: The four most dreadful things in the world are earthquake, thunder, fire, and father. So the Japanese father-son relationship is not the same as the Italian-Mediterranean notion of papa-loves-bambinos. I shall come back to this point at the end. At any rate, it may be safe to say that the competitiveness of Oliver toward his father is a characteristic of the American upper- and upper-middle-class family that is quite unique. I don't know, however, whether Oliver represents a true picture of what really is or whether he is just its caricature. Even if it is caricature, couldn't we say that the competitive spirit portrayed by Oliver sets the tone for all of American society? I don't mean just the business world. It seems to outside observers that it permeates all family relationships, including that of husband and wife. I sometimes wonder if the only relationship which lacks the competitive spirit in this society might be a homosexual one. Or one might mention hippies as new champions to combat the competitive spirit, but, alas, their anticompetitiveness doesn't bring them anywhere near their fathers!

To go back to *Love Story*, a showdown comes when Jenny is forced by Oliver to decline an invitation to his father's sixtieth birthday party. Instead of writing his parents a note about their not coming to the party, as Oliver wanted her to do, Jenny calls Oliver's father, in hopes of at least getting them to talk to each other – something which they haven't done for a long time. Oliver refuses to comply and flares up when she ends the telephone conversation with, 'Mr. Barrett, Oliver does want you to know that in his own special way – Oliver loves you very much.' He rips the phone from her hand, then from the socket, hurls it across the room, and yells at her. But in a moment she disappears, and when he realizes that, he goes out to look for her. He spends the whole day in search for her and comes home exhausted late at night to find her sitting on the doorstep. 'I forgot my key', is her explanation. He blurts out, 'Jenny, I'm sorry –' to which she says, 'Stop!' And she continues in a very quiet voice, 'Love means not ever having to say you're sorry.' After that they don't talk much – no apology, no explanation, no nothing. She says only that she would like to go to sleep. So they both go to bed at once, apparently without even lovemaking, though it is noted that she looks at him reassuringly.

This scene is very interesting. I don't know how ordinary this kind of scene is in American life and whether or not Jenny in this scene is representative of American women. I should think that if she were Japanese, she would have shown at least a trace of self-pity or sulkiness, while if Oliver were Japanese, he would not have said even 'I'm sorry'; certainly he would have shown a great sense of relief and possibly might have spilled out some of his frustrated anger at her. Of course I don't necessarily want to paint Japanese people black. There are nice Japanese, who can control themselves and there are also ill-behaved Americans. In fact it was Oliver who was to blame for the whole chain of events that led up to the scene, and it would be too much to praise him for his apologizing. It surely would have been very odd if he hadn't apologized. But then why does Jenny interrupt his apology and say, 'Love means not ever having to say you're sorry'? Why couldn't she simply accept his apology and be held in his arms, saying something like, 'Oh! I'm sorry, too. I bet you've been looking for me the whole day'?

In this connection let me relate, in passing, some of my observations on the American family. Since I came to the United States years ago for the first time, I have always been struck by the fact that here husbands and wives often say to each other, 'Thank you' or 'I'm sorry'. Americans often speak of Japanese as polite, but I sometimes wonder if in a certain respect Americans are not more polite than Japanese. At any rate, Japanese seldom use expressions like 'Thank you' or 'I'm sorry' within the family or among those with whom they are closely associated. They take each other pretty much for granted and feel that using those phrases would set the members of the family or group apart rather than keeping them close. That is, Japanese feel that the use of words can chill the atmosphere, whereas Americans, in contrast, feel encouraged and reassured by such communication. I think this is clearly related to the psychology of *amae*, because the Japanese idea is that those who are close to each other – that is to say, who are privileged to merge with each other – do not need words to express feelings. One surely would not feel merged with another (that is *amae*), if one had to verbalize a need to do so! On the other hand, Japanese do use those expressions, mainly outside the intimate circle, although even within such a circle one would use them on serious occasions – for instance, when one wants to be forgiven for his misconduct, or when a daughter takes leave of her parents just before her wedding. Interestingly enough, I have come to notice that Americans do not necessarily use those expressions when Japanese do feel that an apology or an expression of gratitude is called for. This of course surprises no one, because the use or non-use of particular verbal formulas is conventional or culturally conditioned. After all, if Americans were always as kind and polite to one another within the family as they appear to be to casual onlookers, there wouldn't be such a high rate of divorce or such violent antagonism between generations in American society.

With this in mind, let us consider how Jenny felt in the face of her family squabble. It is the kind of occurrence which could easily have cooled the couple's affection toward each other, thus paving the way to eventual divorce. In this instance, however, Oliver, being sufficiently mortified, offers her a sincere apology. But then why doesn't she take it? Why does she say, 'Love means not ever having to say you're sorry'? It is not that she rejects his apology, for the two clearly seem to be reconciled to each other. But then what does she mean by that sentence? Was it not that she almost dreaded hearing 'I'm sorry' from him? As if this little phrase could have destroyed the love within her? I think we can surmise what she must have felt after she left the scene of the squabble, what she must have felt while she wandered the streets for hours and while she sat on the doorstep for a long time waiting for him to rescue her from being locked out. Didn't a keen sense of regret over the marriage creep into her mind? It was she who sacrificed a scholarship to study music in France and a career for the marriage and it was she who supported him through school. Didn't she feel that all this was in vain? She must have fought this feeling with all her might. She couldn't afford feeling sorry for herself, as it would have meant a complete defeat to her. One also has to take into account here the fact that Americans have very little capacity for self-pity, but rather hate it enormously. So it may be only natural that she checked her latent inclination to be pitied. His telling her 'I'm sorry' might have touched her sensitive spot, and that is, I believe, why she interrupted his apology.

Here I would like to introduce the Japanese translation of the words: 'Love means not ever having to say you're sorry.' I shall retranslate the Japanese translation of this sentence back into English. It becomes: 'Love means that you never regret.' It completely misses the sense of the original sentence and one may wonder how such a mistranslation could have happened. I don't know myself, since I didn't ask the translator about it. It may simply be an error caused by the carelessness of the translator. But I wonder, if the translator gave an exact rendering of the sentence into Japanese, how meaningful it would sound in Japanese. 'Love means not ever having to say you're sorry.' I have already stated that Japanese seldom use this kind of expression between husband and wife. So, this sentence in Japanese sounds cheap or matter-of-fact, though the original English in the mouth of Jenny could have conveyed something fresh and truly affectionate. One might then say that Jenny was unwittingly striving toward the ideal state of *amae* or the Japanese pattern of husband-and-wife relationship. On the other hand, the sentence 'Love means that you never regret' is forceful in Japanese and makes sense, because Japanese heroines are supposed to not regret their love. The Japanese translation, therefore, matches the weight given to the original sentence in English. Though it is a case of gross mistranslation, one could say that it even gives a better picture of what Jenny might have felt inside, as I suggested a while ago. At any rate, when you go to a Japanese theater where *Love Story* is shown, you see signs everywhere on the wall saying 'Love means that you never regret' in big Japanese characters.

The rest of the story follows the couple through a tragic dénouement, for Jenny gets leukemia and dies. Heroically, Jenny never sinks into self-pity. Instead she tries until the last moment to comfort and strengthen Oliver. On her deathbed she quickly notices the guilty look on Oliver's face and blurts out: 'That guilty look on your face, Oliver, it's sick. . . . It's nobody's fault, you preppie bastard. Would you please *stop* blaming yourself!' Then she continues, 'Screw Paris and music and all the crap you think you stole from me. I don't care, you sonovabitch. Can't you believe that?' I think Jenny felt instinctively that Oliver was like a helpless child who was about to be separated from his loving mother. In terms of the psychology of *amae*, one might say that she responded to his hidden wish for *amae*. But one could also say that she couldn't stand Oliver's feeling guilty, because that would have made her feel sorry for herself and would have broken the sense of unity between the two, which was threatened anyway by her impending death. In other words, she clung desperately to that love which was the only justification for her short life. Now, couldn't this be interpreted as a manifestation of her own repressed wish for *amae*? After all, she was trying to keep the feeling – or to put it more cruelly, the illusion – that she was inseparably one with Oliver. This is indicated quite clearly when as death approaches she begs him to hold her real tight. I think that this kind of love is called romantic in the Western world. I can't here adequately define the meaning of this word, but it seems to me that its important ingredient has to be the feeling of *amae*, as exemplified in the above analysis. For this reason the word 'romantic' quickly became part of the Japanese vocabulary after Japan's initial exposure to Western culture. In fact we have many stories, ancient and new, of the romantic type. I have to admit, however, that Japanese romantic stories are perhaps a bit different from Western ones. For example, if Jenny were Japanese, she wouldn't have used the kind of language she used on her deathbed. I am referring to language of mock aggression, which completely hides Jenny's weakness, yet sufficiently conveys warmth toward Oliver. Japanese women in Jenny's position, as I mentioned above, would and could have betrayed a sense of self-pity, through, for instance, watery eyes, thus inviting pity upon themselves.

Now back to *Love Story*. After Jenny dies, a most curious thing happens. Oliver's father comes to the hospital. Previously, Oliver had gone to him to borrow money for the cost of Jenny's hospitalisation. Oliver had not explained why he needed so much money, but the father had given him the amount he requested. This, incidentally, also impresses me as a proof of the father's great generosity and love toward Oliver; also, the fact that Oliver couldn't tell his father the truth even at this critical moment and that he had to strain himself to say, 'Thank you, Father,' shows again the enormous competitiveness and almost vindictiveness of Oliver toward his father. At any rate, the father must have investigated what was happening to the young couple, and finding out about Jenny's illness, he hurries to the hospital, only to be told at the entrance by Oliver that Jenny is dead, Hearing this, the father says in a stunned whisper, 'I am sorry.' Then something strange happens. Oliver repeats, without knowing why, what he had once heard from Jenny, 'Love means not ever having to say you're sorry.' The next moment he collapses in his father's arms and cries. It is noted that he had never cried in the presence of his father before. What happened? He didn't cry when Jenny died, but cried when his father said the words of condolence to him. Was he finally ready to accept his father's love? I imagine that he might have felt sorry at this moment for the animosity and meanness he had displayed toward his father all these years. But to say 'I'm sorry' at this point was too much for him, and also it was not appropriate for the occasion. So he just repeated the words he had once heard from Jenny, without quite knowing why. In other words, his feeling at this moment could be interpreted as something like this. 'I feel like saying I'm sorry, but since you love me, you wouldn't expect me to say so.' This is, interestingly, identical to what Japanese feel under similar circumstances. I believe that Oliver was able to reconcile himself with his father through the love of Jenny, or, perhaps it would be better to say, through her death.

What is most curious is that this ending was completely cut from the movie version. According to the movie version, the father says to Oliver 'I'm sorry,' but Oliver walks away from his father without even glancing at him and goes out alone to mourn Jenny. Why did the movie cut this ending? Was it because it was too soft? Was it because the American public is not mature enough to appreciate the tender moment of father-son reconciliation? I think it was a grave mistake to cut this ending, because the story concerns the father-son love relationship as much as, if not more than, the young couple's love. When I came to this ending in my reading, I even felt that there was a faint allusion to the famous biblical story of the prodigal son. Was this, then, perhaps why that ending was cut from the movie version – because the contemporary Americans might wish to have nothing to remind them of religion, particularly institutionalized religion? Interestingly, this characterization applies to the couple in the story as well. They were irreligious people and honest ones, too. That is why they refused to have a church wedding. But when they were confronted with the grim reality of Jenny's fatal disease, it is noted that Oliver began to think about God. Not that he was resentful toward God for what was happening to him and to her, but rather because he hoped there was a God that he could thank for still permitting her to remain with him. Wasn't this a precursor of what would happen later – that is, his reconciliation with his father? I think the author showed unusual insight in suggesting a parallel between Oliver's awakening religious thoughts and his eventual reconciliation with his father. And all the more I deplore the fact that the movie version didn't include the whole story.

I have almost exhausted what I can say about *Love Story*, but I would like to add a few more words along the lines of thinking which I have been pursuing so far. Contemporary society is often called a fatherless society. The term, I believe, was first used by Paul Federn and lately has become well known through Mitscherlich's book which uses the term as its title. I shall not go into details here of what these learned men think about our contemporary fatherless society. I would only like to mention the curious fact that in spite of their clamor for the downfall of authority and establishment, the youngsters seem to be wishing to see a strong and dependable father figure emerge. Take Oliver as an example. He fought his father fiercely, almost killed him in fantasy, yet there was a hidden tender spot in him which yearned for his father. I know that many Western people feel that the Japanese father-son relationship is different from Oliver's case, that in Japan sons must always be respectful and obedient toward their fathers. This is a stereotyped notion, however, and it seems to me to bespeak a projection on the part of Western people. In other words, they perhaps want to believe that somewhere in the world people still truly respect their fathers. Thus, the fact that a good many Western intellectuals flock to Oriental mysticism or religion could be interpreted as a search for a missing father figure or a God they killed in their hearts. But alas, their efforts will be wasted, because they will not find in those esoteric exercises what they are really searching for. I think at least some of them now realize that dabbling with Oriental mysticism is getting them nowhere. Perhaps that is why they drug themselves, in their frantic search for something.

Then, what is the father-son relationship really like in Japan? If Japanese do not fight the father the way Oliver does, how do they treat him? How do they live with him? To explain this, I shall again have recourse to the story of the prodigal son, this time the case of the older brother who never left the father. Was he happy living with the father? No. When the father welcomed home the younger brother who had spent all his money in debauchery, the older brother said, 'Look, all these years I have slaved for you and never once disobeyed your orders, yet you never offered me so much as a kid for me to celebrate with my friends.' So, in the older brother's eyes, the father's welcome of the younger brother only seemed to be one more instance of the father's being capricious, unpredictable, and tyrannical. The older brother was close to the father physically, but in his heart was far away from him. To him, there was no loving father. And I should say that this is the way many Japanese feel about their fathers. Couldn't we say, then, that in a way Japanese society is also fatherless? Fathers in Japanese society play the role of breadwinner all right, but they usually spend very little time with the family. Hence they seldom, interact with children, and when they do, they usually do so through mothers. There are occasions when they make their presence felt directly, but then they tend to act like natural elements – like earthquake, thunder or fire – that is, very frighteningly, as the saying mentioned above indicates.

I think it would be useful for Western people to realize, since we are getting into closer and closer contact with each other, that there are, roughly speaking, two ways of relating to a father, yours and ours. Oliver is you, so you can understand him. You can leave father, can live a life free of father – at least you think you can. Then you impose your way of life, intentionally or unintentionally, upon non-Western people, often in the name of democracy or modernization. But don't forget that they might take you as father instead – capricious, unpredictable, and tyrannical at that! Even if they consent to live under your roof, under your umbrella of protection, and seem to enjoy dependency, there might be a smoldering resentment in time. I imagine, for instance, that is what many Japanese became acutely aware of when President Nixon suddenly announced behind their backs his plan to visit China. I am afraid that in veering from *Love Story* into international politics I am going astray, but truly all these cross-cultural thoughts have been stimulated in me by the story.

REFERENCES

Doi, L. Takeo. '*Amae* – A Key Concept for Understanding Japanese Personality Structure', in R. J. Smith and R. K. Beardsley (Eds.), *Japanese Culture: Its Development and Characteristics*; Aldine, 1962.

Doi, L. Takeo. 'Some Thoughts on Helplessness and the Desire To Be Loved', *Psychiatry* (1963) 26:266-272.

Doi, L. Takeo. 'Psychoanalytic Therapy and "Western Man": A Japanese View', *Internat. J. Social Psychiatry* (1964) Special Ed. No. 1 (Congress Issue), pp. 13-18.

Federn, Paul. 'On the Psychology of Revolution: The Fatherless Society' [1919], trans. Rudolf Ekstein; *Reiss-Davis Clinic Bull.* (1971) 8(1) :11-33.

Mitscherlich, Alexander. *Society Without the Father*, trans. E. Mosbach; Harcourt, Brace & World, 1969.

Segal, Erich. *Love Story*; Signet, 1970.

First published in *Bulletin of the Menninger Clinic*, Vol.37, No.2, March 1973

⑪ Psychotherapy as 'Hide-and-Seek' *

I want to propose a theoretical model which fits all kinds of psychotherapy, ancient and modern, East and West. It is a deceptively simple idea: *the essence of psychotherapy in any form is 'hide-and-seek'*.

Hide-and-seek is probably the most primitive, hence the most international children's game. Because it is so elementary, the books on children's games do not describe it. Interestingly enough, Eric Berne, who wrote the famous book, *Games People Play*, did not mention it either. It must have eluded his discerning eyes (to put it ironically) because it was the very game he was playing professionally.

However, one even more primitive game of disappearing-reappearing, called *inai-inai-bah* in Japanese, is not actually a children's game, for adults have to engage infants to play it. For instance, the mother hides her face saying '*inai-inai*', which means 'now gone', and then shows her face saying '*bah!*' – a special exclamation which means 'here now'. The repetition of these two acts invariably elicits a smile in the infant, a phenomenon which indicates (in psychoanalytic terms) that the infant has beginning object relations. The infant then comes to learn the trick and immensely enjoys trying it himself on the adult. Japanese parents may engage the child in this play from a very early age, even five months, and perhaps other nationalities also have a similar game. Peek-a-boo is one example, although the emphasis here is not upon the repetition of disappearing-reappearing, but upon the sudden appearance of a familiar face; hence its onset must be later than *inai-inai-bah*.

A play of *fort-da* by a little boy of one and a half observed by Freud (1920) has definitely the theme of disappearing-reappearing. 'The child had a wooden reel with a piece of string tied round it. . . . What he did was to hold the reel by the string and very skilfully throw it over the edge of his curtained cot, letting it disappear into it, at the same time uttering his expressive '*o-o-o-o*'. He then pulled the reel out of the cot again by the string and hailed its reappearance with the joyful "*da*".' According to Freud's interpretation, the little boy apparently made into play his experiences of letting his mother go, only to see her come back later.

---

* Presented at the Conference on Culture and Mental Health in Asia and the Pacific, March 19-25, 1972, Honolulu, Hawaii, and published in the Proceedings of that Conference. Reprinted by permission of University of Hawaii Press.

This, then, was a solitary game invented by one particular boy. At any rate, what interests me is the fact that the disappearing-reappearing game, or something like it, seems to be a precursor of hide-and-seek; there is a developmental continuum from the disappearing-reappearing game to hide-and-seek.

In abstract terms, one could say that the game of hide-and-seek involves two activities: secret formation and its discovery. So it presupposes a certain level of psychological development, which in my observations includes a capacity for a kind of lying. This should not be equated with delinquent lying, however; rather it is innocent lying for the sake of preserving one's separate self. For instance, suppose a child does not want to be reminded by his mother every morning to wash his face, so one morning he said he did when he did not.

To put this situation into psychoanalytic terms once again, one can only say that those who have reached the oedipal stage can and will play hide-and-seek. Hence, a too young child who is made to play the game often announces himself from a hiding place and, if forced to play the role of seeking others in hiding, he is likely to cry or give up playing unless the others make it easy for him to find them. He is still fixed to the stage of the disappearing-reappearing game. Incidentally, Japanese call the role of seeker *oni*. This word is usually translated as 'demon', but it may refer to the person who for one reason or another isolates himself from society, that is, the alienated one. So, it is appropriate that the one who was first discovered in hide-and-seek, that is, the one who lost the game, becomes *oni*. In English, *oni* is referred to simply as 'it'. I wonder if this appellative carries the same feeling as *oni*. Perhaps it does.

When I say that the essence of psychotherapy is 'hide-and-seek', it is because the patient is induced to look for the secret of his illness by the therapist. The patient can be thought of as a frustrated and lost *oni*, and the therapist comes to help him. But since the secret of his illness, which they work together to find, lies hidden in the patient himself, the psychotherapeutic 'hide-and-seek' is really played within the person of the patient. That is why it is so difficult to find and why he needs the therapist's help. Sometimes it might appear that the therapist is the real *oni*, and the patient is the one who tries to escape the therapist's attention. Or the patient might act like *oni* toward the therapist and wish to pursue the therapist's secrets. Still, if the patient is within the neurotic range, he can be easily interested in finding out the secret of his illness. But, if he is psychotic, it is hard to engage him in the psychotherapeutic 'hide-and-seek'. He is either in no mood to play the game or he is feeling terrified because he is convinced his 'secrets' are out, that is, he feels exposed and defenseless. In such a case, one may say he is literally *oni*, the alienated one not interested in playing the game. The therapist then has to bolster up the patient's ego and try to posit the patient's secrets within himself again.

This formulation of psychotherapy in terms of 'hide-and-seek' seems to apply best to psychoanalytic therapy. After all, it was Freud himself who tried to discover the secret of neurosis. He became convinced he succeeded in this search, thus bequeathing his personal experiences to posterity in the form of psychoanalytic therapy. However, I wonder if the above formulation cannot be applied to other kinds of psychotherapy, too, even though what is thought of as the secret of neurosis must differ according to various schools. But the sense of a secret and its discovery may not be so pronounced in other schools as in Freudian psychoanalysis.

ORIENTAL PSYCHOTHERAPIES

In shamanistic therapies the secret is, of course, what a shaman divines. In Morita therapy the secret is the patient's *toraware*, meaning the state of being bound up with one's physical and mental conditions which, in the last analysis, is attributed to the self-preservative instinct. In actual therapy the patient is supposed to develop insight into and, at the same time, transcend his *toraware* by engaging in various occupations within a setting of communal living. For Naikan, the secret is one's unconfessed sins or unacknowledged indebtedness and, here again, the therapeutic process takes place in a setting of communal living.

I believe the therapeutic use of communal living is characteristic of Japanese psychotherapies. Also, it should be noted that the emphasis in Japanese psychotherapies is laid not so much upon seeking out a hidden secret as upon rescuing the trapped, hidden person and luring him back to communal living. One may say then that in these therapies the psychotherapeutic 'hide-and-seek' is heavily slanted toward the disappearing-reappearing game.

Along with this change in emphasis, one can also see a subtle shifting in the meaning of 'secret', because what strikes the patient as well as the therapist as 'secret' is not really one's inner secrets, but what makes man transcend them. In other words, the therapy itself becomes shrouded with the sense of secret, or perhaps better, mystery. This point, of course, is more pronounced in all religiously-inspired therapies or healing cults, not only Japanese, but other nationalities as well.

In this connection, it may be relevant to point out that for the awakening infant the object is always something wonderous or even mysterious. That is why he can be delighted by *inai-inai-bah* or peek-a-boo. This is not to maintain, however, that the sense of wonder or mystery is just infantile. After all, both philosophy and religion may owe their origin to it. In this regard one may recall the famous words of Aristotle that wonder is the instigator of philosophical endeavor and, in the Old Testament, the frequent references to the face of Yahweh. Etymologically interesting is the fact the Japanese word *himitsu*, which was originally coined as a Buddhistic term, can signify both secret and mystery (like the German word *Geheimnis*), though nowadays it refers more often to secret, as its Buddhistic meaning has become almost lost.

It is a known fact that psychoanalytic therapy has never caught the fancy of the Japanese people. Without meaning to disparage them, one may compare them to small children who are reluctant to play hide-and-seek. It is not that they are not troubled by inner secrets, rather they are often greatly troubled, since inner secrets hinder them from satisfactory communal living. But they are not interested in finding out about their inner secrets. They only wish to get rid of them and, if they cannot, they pretend they have no secrets. They seem to behave like the small children who, still being fixed at the stage of the disappearing-reappearing game, come out from hiding in order to be found and, if nobody comes to find them, they become grieved.

This argument is essentially the one I expounded in another paper (1964). Using the concept of *amae*, I stated that Japanese who tend to value dependence, and shy away from the dichotomy of subject and object, will not warm up to psychoanalytic therapy as it is practiced in the West. However, there is an element of the disappearing-reappearing game in psychoanalytic therapy itself called transference; though, according to the rule, this phenomenon also has to be analyzed eventually, that is, to be identified for its real nature. In other words, in psychoanalytic therapy it is assumed that the disappearing-reappearing play has to be resolved into 'hide-and-seek'.

Japanese as children play hide-and-seek, and there is no reason why they cannot play the psychotherapeutic 'hide-and-seek' if they are skilfully encouraged to do so. In this regard, the activity of creating secrets and their discovery constitute the antipode to *amae*. Whereas *amae* represents the desire to merge with others, to cultivate or pursue secrets leads rather to the establishment of one's separate self and the mastery of the world. It is not that Japanese lack the native inclination for the latter activities; it seems they have not given free rein to them for some historical or sociological reason.

IMPLICATIONS FOR PSYCHOTHERAPY

Finally a few words about the climate of the present age and its implications for psychotherapy. We know that people everywhere in the world are now having the curious feeling of being driven out from their hiding places. This phenomenon is undoubtedly related to the fact that the natural habitat of man is being destroyed rapidly by the enormously accelerated advance of technology. The outward changes are matched by the changes in man's inner world since it now seems that every secret not only of nature but of man and society as well is made bare. I think the unmasking trend in literature, which began in 19th Century Europe and spread over the whole world, has greatly contributed to this outcome along with the advances made in every field of science. Interestingly and significantly, sex no longer spells secrecy in our contemporary society. In such an atmosphere it would be extremely difficult to play 'hide-and-seek', because the ordinary man feels as exposed and denuded as psychotics. Man then hankers for mystery anew or tries to create artificial secrets, as can be seen by the recent rise of interest in occultism, mysticism, mystery stories, and political secrets.

I think the fact that psychoanalytic therapy is not now in such vogue even in the West as it used to be is related to this change in the mental climate of the age, although it is an irony that such change may be at least partly due to psychoanalysis itself, that is, the dissemination of psychoanalytic knowledge among the public. As a result, contemporary man would rather engage in the disappearing-reappearing play than in the psychotherapeutic 'hide-and-seek'. This fact helped create, I think, two apparently unrelated opposite effects. One is the search for some effective therapy which promises to rescue man from the modem predicament – hence the renewed interest in all kinds of brief therapy like crisis intervention, encounter therapy or sensitivity training and also traditional folk therapy. The other is that psychoanalytic therapy, if it is undertaken nowadays, tends to be a long, drawn-out business stretched over many years, inasmuch as man gets easily stuck with the disappearing-reappearing play which is its legitimate ingredient.

REFERENCES

Doi, L. Takeo: Psychoanalytic Therapy and 'Western Man' – A Japanese View. *Int. J. Soc. Psychiat.*, Special Edition No. 1 (Congress Issue), 1964, pp. 13-18.
Freud, Sigmund (1920): Beyond the Pleasure Principle. *Standard Edition* 18:14-16, 1955.

First published in *The Quarterly Journal of Speech*, Vol.59, No.2, pp. 180-185, April 1973

⑫ The Japanese Patterns of Communication and the Concept of *Amae*

The first paper in which I introduced the concept of *amae* appeared in an American speech journal, the 1956 Spring issue of *Western Speech*, under the title of 'Japanese Language as an Expression of Japanese Psychology'. This came about because Professor Don Geiger, the editor of the Journal at that time, was a good friend of mine. Actually he and another friend of mine, Professor Anthony Ostroff, both of the University of California in Berkeley, helped me considerably when I prepared the paper for the convention of the American Psychiatric Association in the fall of 1955. They showed great interest in what I had to say, and that is why my paper ended up in a speech journal instead of a psychiatric journal.

I think some of you are already familiar with the concept of *amae*, but for those who are not I shall first quote the relevant passage from the above-mentioned paper:

> *Amaeru* [*amae* is its noun form] can be translated as 'to depend and presume upon another's love'. This word has the same root as *amai*, an adjective which corresponds to 'sweet'. Thus *amaeru* has a distinct feeling of sweetness, and is generally used to express a child's attitude toward an adult, especially his parents. I can think of no English word equivalent to *amaeru* except for 'spoil', which, however, is a transitive verb and definitely has a bad connotation; whereas the Japanese *amaeru* does not necessarily have a bad connotation, although we say we should not let a youngster *amaeru* too much. I think most Japanese adults have a dear memory of the taste of sweet dependency as a child and, consciously or unconsciously, carry a lifelong nostalgia for it (p. 92).

Thus it is true that *amaeru* has its primary locus in childhood, but it can be applied to any interpersonal relationship between adults, if that is known to contain the same kind of longing for dependency or belonging as a child must have. It dawned on me then that the visibility or accessibility of such a basic desire as *amae* might be the very factor that distinguishes Japanese people from other nations. So I wrote '*Amae* – A Key Concept for Understanding Japanese Personality Structure',[1] when I was asked to participate in the symposium on culture and personality, a program of the Tenth Pacific Science Congress held in Honolulu in 1961. In this paper I stressed the central importance of *amae* for the Japanese patterns of emotion, which seemed to find a linguistic confirmation in the existence of a rich vocabulary in the Japanese language centering around the theme of *amae* with its multifarious shades. I argued that this fact must be indicative of the characteristics of Japanese society, that in Japan parental dependency is fostered and its behavior pattern institutionalized into the social structure. Today I am not going to elaborate upon the structural aspect of Japanese society that bears out *amae*, the area which should be better reserved for Prof. Nakane to discuss. Instead I shall try to demonstrate how the psychology of *amae* pervades and actually makes the Japanese patterns of communication.

Let me state at the beginning that the existence of the rich vocabulary centering around the theme of *amae* indicates foremost the awareness, not the fulfilment, on the part of Japanese people of the all-powerful desire to *amaeru*. They of course would like to gratify such a desire if they can, but since this is not always feasible, they have to develop a special sensitivity as to when and where they can gratify it and a capacity to endure the painful frustrations that would invariably occur. In other words, the rich vocabulary concerning *amae* attests to the appreciation of dependency needs in Japanese society as well as to the attempt at controlling such needs. Surely such controlling mechanisms are called for, for the desire to *amaeru* is entirely contingent upon others for its gratification. Namely, one cannot conjure its gratification by a verbal magic as sometimes can be done in the case of 'I love you'. In fact, Japanese seldom say 'I *amaeru* on you', though they may say something like that when they are much obliged. Still, the gratification of *amaeru* stands as the norm in Japanese society, or perhaps it is better to say, as the principle of mutuality which alone guarantees a smooth transaction.

This being so, suppose that all inter-personal communications in Japanese society have the emotional undertone of *amae*. Then, would it be surprising that Japanese tend to have many short breaks in their conversation? Apparently during those breaks they try to feel out one another and assess the situation. Because what is most important for Japanese is to reassure themselves on every occasion of a mutuality based upon *amae*. One could say then that for Japanese verbal communication is something that accompanies non-verbal communication and not the other way around. In other words, they are very sensitive to the atmosphere pervading human relationships. Either they will try to soften the atmosphere or they are afraid to spoil it. No wonder that they often look pensive, smile unnaturally, at any rate are not properly communicative; the vices of which Japanese are often accused by foreign observers.

To explain this point further, let me introduce to you a very interesting comparative research done by Dr. William Caudill and Mrs. Helen Weinstein. They selected a matched sample of 30 Japanese and 30 American three-to-four months-old infants and studied the interactions of those infants with their mothers. The conclusion the authors draw from this study is astounding:

> American infants are more happily vocal, more active, and more
> exploratory of their bodies and their physical environment, than are
> Japanese infants. Directly related to these findings, the American mother is
> in greater vocal interaction with her infant, and stimulates him to greater
> physical activity and exploration. The Japanese mother, in contrast, is in
> greater bodily contact with her infant, and soothes him toward physical
> quiescence, and passivity with regard to his environment. Moreover, these
> patterns of behavior, so early learned by the infant, are in line with the
> differing expectations for late behavior in the two cultures as the child
> grows to be an adult.[2]

One can see easily from this that Americans are conditioned from the very
beginning of life to associate human contact with verbal communication,
whereas Japanese, more with nonverbal empathic communication.

In this connection I would like to tell you my first reaction to Americans
when I went to the United States in 1950. I was greatly surprised, almost
perturbed by the fact that Americans love to talk incessantly whenever they
get together, even during the meal. As a matter of fact, they sounded to me
almost hypomanic. This impression was undoubtedly at least partly due to
the language barrier I was then painfully aware of, partly due to the
difference in customs between the United States and Japan; because, when
we were growing up, we used to be chided if we chatted during the meal.
But I thought there was more to it, for I could not help feeling that
Americans hate silence, whereas Japanese can sit together comfortably
without saying a word to one another. To tell you the truth, even though I
no longer feel the pinch of the language barrier now, it is still a strain for me
to keep pace with Americans during a social evening. I cannot hide behind
the couch so to speak, as when I am acting professionally. At any rate, I
often bless myself for being a psychiatrist because of the privilege of
keeping silence except for occasional 'wise' comments!

One more example to prove the point. I know one Japanese
simultaneous interpreter who recently served at three international
conferences held in Tokyo and Kyoto. He told me it was simply amazing
that Japanese participants did not communicate much vis-à-vis Americans.
I remind you that they didn't have to speak English, as they could count on
the ample service of simultaneous interpreters. Still, according to my
informant, they didn't talk much, looking most of the time stiff and stony-
faced. Don't think that they were simply awed by the presence of dignified
Americans, though this might have played a role. Because Japanese don't
talk much even at conferences of Japanese only, this even when they are
congenial with one another. They usually spend a long time fishing for
clues as to where each of them stands on the question at issue, so that they
can somehow reach unanimous agreement, which they are so eager to have
on any occasion.

Speaking of unanimous agreement, it has a very important social
function for Japanese. It is a token that the mutuality of all the members
has been preserved. In other words, it is a token satisfaction of *amae*. For
Japanese hate to contradict or to be contradicted, that is, to have to say 'no'

in the intercourse. Since they don't want to have divided opinions in the first place, if such an outcome turns out to be inevitable, they get so heated and emotional that it becomes almost impossible to have reasoned discussions. I think this explains why the Japanese Diet or any intra-group strife in Japan becomes violent. The greater the power of cohesiveness, the more violent the effect of breaking up. It is like splitting the atom.

Now the well-known Japanese fondness for hesitation or ambiguities of expression can also be explained along the same line. Japanese hesitate or say something ambiguous when they fear that what they have in mind might be disagreeable to others, that is to say, when they have to say no. To impress you how deeply ingrained this trait runs in Japanese people from immemorial time let me cite from *Manyoshu*, the oldest anthology of Japanese poems, composed in the eighth century. The story behind the poems in question is as follows: A beautiful girl was sued by two boys, who fought fiercely over her. She apparently could not let her mind be known as to whom she loved, and lamenting for the fact that a humble maid as she was, she became the cause of two boys' fight, she killed herself. Hearing the death of the girl, one of the two boys at once killed himself and the other left behind was much grieved that the one who at once followed her to death might have beaten him. He couldn't swallow his defeat, however, so he killed himself also soon after. The villagers deeply mourned over the deaths of three young people and built monumental mounds for each with the one for the girl in the middle. Several years passed. The tree planted in front of the girl's mound stretched its branch toward one of the other two mounds. The villagers then said, 'Now we know for sure which of the two the girl loved, as the tree stretched its branch.' Please note in this story that there is no condemnation of suicide, nor of the girl's apparent indecisiveness. If anything, she is appreciated for having been so modest and tenderhearted that she could not bear seeing two boys fighting over her. This is Japanese! I have been told that nowhere else in world literature is found such a story, horrendous yet very moving.

Concerning the Japanese ambiguity I have more things to say. That the Japanese language is so constructed as to be particularly conducive to the effect of ambiguity is well known. For instance, Japanese verbs come at the end of the sentence. Therefore, unless and until you hear the whole sentence, you wouldn't know where the speaker stands. This apparently gives him a psychological advantage, as he can change his position in anticipation of your possible reaction to it. However, it may happen that you are often left wondering whether he really means what he says. Also, there is the case of numerous auxiliary words in the Japanese language which primarily function as adhesives of other words and sentences. Since I am not a student of the Japanese grammar, I cannot adequately explain them except that they roughly correspond to conjunctives, interjections, or auxiliary verbs in English. Contrary to English, however, those Japanese equivalents have a very unique feature of faithfully reflecting the speaker's reaction to the changing situation. That is why we can do without pronouns in everyday conversation, a fact which may occasion ambiguity at times. Other factors, too, create ambiguity. Take conjunctives, for instance. In English they provide logical connections. Not necessarily so in Japanese. Rather, more often they serve only to cement and induce the speaker's free associations. At the same time they may help to hold the audience's attention. So, whether spoken or written, Japanese communication is usually quite loose in logical connections. You can go on talking for hours, even gracefully, without coming to the point. That is why it is sometimes extremely difficult to render a Japanese speech or article into English.

The Japanese fondness for unanimous agreement may also contribute to the effect of ambiguity. Curious as it may seem, for Japanese the form of unanimous agreement is not strictly binding, even if obligatory to respect it, which in itself, I am afraid, is an ambiguous statement. What I mean is this. Since the unanimous agreement is a token that the mutuality of all the members has been preserved, it is all right as long as one does not openly challenge its being a *fait accompli*. In other words, it doesn't prevent individual members from harboring their own thoughts or feelings. Here comes the famous Japanese double standard of *tatemae* and *honne*. The former can be translated as 'principle' and the latter 'true mind'. But all of this is rather misleading. Because it looks then as though Japanese espouse hypocrisy as their morality, which is not at all the case. *Tatemae* is any rule of conduct which Japanese accept by unanimous agreement and it would be wrong if you think that Japanese don't take it seriously. It is like a valuable license that secures them membership in a coveted group. Still it is a formal front rather than a principle, behind which one may safely and continuously entertain one's *honne*. The discrepancy between the two is born, if not so bravely, with a good conscience. So for Japanese themselves there is nothing ambiguous about the double standard of *tatemae* and *honne*. It is even quite rational, as it seems that this is the only way things can be done given the nature of Japanese society. As a matter of fact, it is deemed the measure of maturity in Japan to acknowledge the existence of such a double standard and to adjust one's life accordingly. Incidentally, the distinction between *tatemae* and *honne* corresponds in the Japanese mind to the distinction between the public and the private, a topic which Professor Barnlund has taken up this morning.[3] These two pairs of concepts, however, are not really the same. This should be clear, if you trace historically the meanings given to the public or the private.

I am wondering if I have succeeded so far in making the Japanese patterns of communication intelligible to you. If I have, then hopefully you will find the notorious Japanese ambiguity no longer annoying. Writing this paper, I often fancied its title to be 'In Defense of the Japanese Ambiguity', if not 'In Praise of the Japanese Ambiguity'. Of course I am not defending ambiguity as such. I am only saying that ambiguity has a meaning. Only if we know it, ambiguity disappears for all practical purposes. But if we don't, ambiguity may even increase. Such a result is likely to happen when and where two cultures meet. That is, ambiguity in a foreign culture is not appreciated for its hidden meaning, instead is condemned in the name of one's own culture, thus making it even more difficult to understand. I think such danger is particularly great for Japanese culture, for it abounds in ambiguity, even makes a virtue of it as can be seen from its moral code, as I hinted above, or its cultivation of Zen Buddhism or its literary sensibility of which the best example is *haiku*. Unfortunately, nowadays it is not just foreigners who misunderstand Japanese culture, but Japanese as well who fall under the spell of Western ideas. So one may see many Japanese youth denouncing the double standard of *tatemae* and *honne* as adult hypocrisy to the great consternation of the older generation.

Only if they know what they are doing! Because it seems to me that they really don't know either Japanese culture or Western culture. They are only mixing up two cultures and getting mixed up themselves as a result. Please note that I am not just trying to save Japanese culture from contamination by Western culture. Intercultural communication is here to stay, and I shall be doomed if I fight it. I am only saying that for intercultural communication to be really fruitful each culture has to be understood from its roots. To get back to Japanese youth who feel compelled to denounce their own tradition, first they have to rediscover Japanese culture within themselves. Then they have to study Western culture more objectively. For instance, do they know why Western idealism, either in the form of democracy or communism, insists that the ideal is something that can be truly realized on this earth? It is so different from the concept of *tatemae*. Where does that belief come from? It is only because of this belief that one who does not live up to one's professed ideal is denounced as hypocritical. Or perhaps in the latter-day West is this belief being undermined? So much so that Western people do not suffer from the sense of guilt as they used to and have acquired the sense of being realistic. But then, isn't this contemporary sense of being realistic, which is not related at all to the original meaning of realism either in philosophy, literature or fine arts, similar to the Japanese double standard of *tatemae* and *honne*? If so, what does it mean, since they couldn't have borrowed it from Japan? Would it be rather that what appears to be peculiarly Japanese is really a universal human trait and Western people came to appreciate it only at this late date?

I am afraid I am going astray into a much too complicated matter. But this is the kind of thing we have to tackle, if we want seriously to engage in intercultural communication. Only going through such a difficult path, I am convinced, may we be able to create a truly integrated world culture out of the present chaos brought about by too rash intercultural communication.

NOTES

L. Takeo Doi is Professor of Mental Health at the University of Tokyo. This paper was first presented at the 1972 Summer Conference on Intercultural Communication at International Christian University in Tokyo, July 9 to 17.

1.   In *Japanese Culture: Its Development and Characteristics*, ed. Robert J. Smith and Richard K. Beardsley, Viking Fund Publication in Anthropology, No. 34 (New York, 1962), pp. 132-239.

2.   'Maternal Care and Infant Behavior in Japan and America', *Psychiatry*, 32 (Feb. 1969), 42.

3.   *Editor's Note*: Dean Barnlund's study of these concepts in Japan will soon be published in Japanese. (*The Public and Private Self in Japan and The United States*, Tokyo: Simul Press.) Publication in English has not yet been arranged.

First published in the *Journal of Nervous and Mental Disease.* © The Williams and Wilkins Co. USA. Vol.157, No.4, 1973

⑬ *Omote* and *Ura*: Concepts Derived from the Japanese Two-fold Structure of Consciousness

The implications for Japanese psychological functioning of the inter-relationships of two concepts familiar to Japanese are discussed: *omote*, literally 'face' is the pattern one would show to others; *ura*, 'mind' in old Japanese, those private and intimate thoughts which generally are not to be shown to others.

Bill Caudill and I met for the first time in 1954, when he was having his first Japanese experiences and I was groping to formulate my clinical experiences in terms of what I learned in America. Subsequent years made us real comrades in arms, since I served as a consultant to his research in Japan and he was a most appreciative audience as I was developing my own thinking. I was much encouraged because he so often cited my work in his papers and I wrote many papers in English thanks to his support. We even produced one joint paper, 'Interrelations of Psychiatry, Culture and Emotion in Japan',[1] which summarized some of our congruent viewpoints and findings. What follows now has been written as an extension of our long collaborative work. I think Bill would have approved of my saying this with his characteristic understanding smile.

Let me first explain the title of this paper, for the readers may wonder at once what is so unique about the two-fold or even multifold structure of consciousness. Doesn't everyone have some things that he wants to keep to himself or to confide only to someone very close? The front he presents to the public eye is often different from what he thinks he is. According to William James (p. 294) 'a man has as many social selves as there are individuals who recognize him and carry an image of him in their mind'. All this is certainly true, and I acknowledge that what I call the Japanese two-fold structure of consciousness is essentially a universal human trait. Only I want to say that this trait is cultivated to an unusual extent in Japan so that it has come to represent a definite pattern of living. Hence, the need to use special concepts to describe it.

These concepts are conveyed by two Japanese words, *omote* and *ura*, which Japanese use to indicate the contrasting attitudes in dealing with social situations. These words, like the English equivalents 'front' and 'rear', literally refer to the fore and back sides of things. Apart from this literal use, however, they are sometimes used in naming things to suggest the social function of the thing thus named. For instance, *omote-guchi* (front-door) is the main entrance to Japanese houses which is of use for the members of a family or their guests, but the maid or the shopmen who call either to take orders or to deliver things use only *ura-guchi* (kitchen-door). *Omote-dori* or *omote-kaido* is a busy street and *ura-dori* or *ura-kaido* a lonely alley, hence these two words may be used to imply a success or the lack of it. As can be seen from these usages, *omote* is the appearance one would show to others. In this it is interesting to note that *omote* means 'face' and *ura* 'mind' in old literary Japanese. That one is able to build up *omote* is a commendable thing in Japan. It means that one is finally on one's own. It is different from a similar English expression, 'to put up a front', which has the bad connotation of making a show. *Ura* is the reverse of *omote*, that is, what one would hide from others. Hence, to take *ura* (*ura o kaku*) is to attack from behind. To cut *ura* (*uragiru*) is to betray. That *ura* aches (*urayamu*) is to envy. It is also used as prefix to some adjectives, such as *ura-ganashii* (sad), *ura-sabishii* (lonely), to indicate that one who so feels cannot identify its cause.

Thus, when Japanese say the affairs of *omote* (*omote no hanashi*), they mean what they do in order to impress others whose presence puts them on guard. Conversely, when they say the matters of *ura* (*ura-no hanashi*), they mean their secrets which they will disclose only to those who are closest to them. These two might contradict each other in substance, but that doesn't matter to Japanese. Furthermore, when one is in the state of *omote*, *omote* is everything and *ura* virtually does not exist for him. Likewise, when one is in *ura*, one can forget about the existence of *omote*. Only one should be able to discern which is the time for *omote* and which for *ura*. The ease with which one shifts from *omote* to *ura* and back again without much strain is regarded as the measure of one's social maturity. In other words, it doesn't blemish a man's integrity to take recourse to one or the other depending upon the particular situation he finds himself in. Rather his integrity rests upon the complete mastery of *omote* and *ura*.

In this connection I would like to introduce two more Japanese words, *tatemae* and *honne*. *Tatemae* is a certain formal principle which is palatable to everybody concerned so that the harmony of a group is guaranteed, while *honne* is the feelings or opinions which they privately hold regarding the matter. It is admitted that there may be an apparent discrepancy between the two, yet they are supposed to coexist in peace. It must be clear from this explanation that the relationship of *tatemae* to *honne* is the same as that of *omote* to *ura*. As a matter of fact, *tatemae* and *honne* can perhaps best be defined as the *omote*-mind and the *ura*-mind respectively. Japanese evidently need both. The two are complementary to each other. Literally there is no *omote* (front) without *ura* (rear) and no *ura* without *omote*. Likewise, *tatemae* doesn't stand alone without tacit support from *honne* and the latter cannot be entertained without the former's protection.

Why do Japanese make much of the distinction between *omote* and *ura*, that is the distinction between what can be shown to others and what cannot and elevate it to a rule of daily living? I think this is definitely related to the psychology of *amae* that prevails in Japanese society, which I explained in a number of articles.[2-4] *Amae* is a dependency need which manifests itself in a longing to merge with others. This longing can be fulfilled under satisfactory conditions in infancy, but surely it cannot be easily fulfilled as one grows up. But if *amae* is set forth as the principle of a society regulating the smooth transactions of its members, wouldn't that society have to institute a certain token indicating that this need is taken care of? I think that is what happened in Japanese society. Namely, *omote* or *tatemae* is a token that the mutuality of members of a group is preserved, while *ura* or *honne* which acknowledges the inevitable frustrations in *amae* is given free rein as long as it does not dispute the former. This is surely a very ingenious way of handling ambivalent feelings. The fact that Japanese frequently exchange gifts saying, 'This is only *oshirushi* (token) of my gratitude (or apology)', is definitely related to this. It also explains why Japanese look so homogeneous and cohesive, yet if and when no *tatemae* is available why they so easily resort to violence.

The above description of the Japanese two-fold structure of consciousness might give an impression that it is after all a double standard of morality. This impression is perhaps strongest among foreigners who have to make a certain deal with Japanese. They of course do not share the same values with Japanese. What Japanese present them as *omote* or *tatemae* sounds to them like empty words. So they complain that Japanese are shrewd and vain in spite of their apparent politeness and sincerity, that Japanese are too fond of formalities even in social intercourse and seldom reveal what they really think and feel. I should maintain, however, that Japanese do not espouse the double standard of morality deliberately. Rather it is truer to say that they are driven toward it because of their cultural heritage, as I explained above. Furthermore, at times Japanese themselves may find it unhappy to behave in *omote* or *ura* alternately. In fact, to learn how to do it is a growing pain for every Japanese child. For many adults the pain they incurred as a child ensues in the permanent splitting of their ego. They cannot integrate *omote* and *ura* adequately. Hence, they envy and extoll a person who appears to have no splitting of *omote* and *ura* and hate intensely anybody who makes use of such splitting to promote his selfish interest.

I think that the famous Japanese fondness of nature can also be understood from the same angle. For Japanese must feel greatly relieved with nature since they don't have to play *omote* and *ura* with it. They become one with nature so to speak and can indulge in the feeling of pure *amae*. From their viewpoint therefore they feel more human with nature than with humans. Lest it be thought, however, that I maintain that an attitude toward nature is only peculiarly Japanese, let me quote a few lines from William Wordsworth's *Tintern Abbey Revisited*, which seem to echo exactly the same feelings:

> . . . well pleased to recognize
> In Nature and the language of the sense,
> The anchor of my purest thoughts, the muse,
> The guide, the guardian of my heart and soul
> Of all my moral being . . .
> Knowing that Nature never did betray
> The heart that loved her.

So such fond feelings for nature are not exclusively Japanese, though it may be said that they are much more pronounced and pervasive in Japan. In fact Japan had not just one Wordsworth, but hundreds and thousands like him who gave expression to those feelings. One would argue further that even Wordsworth was too discursive compared with the total immersion of Japanese in nature. So far so good. But this main relationship Japanese have with nature has one basic defect: It doesn't teach Japanese how to protect and spare nature. That is, I believe, why they did practically nothing to prevent the vast destruction wrought upon nature in recent years. It could happen in spite of their extreme fondness of nature, or, to put it ironically, perhaps because of it.

Finally, I should like to mention one general usage of the concepts *omote* and *ura*, though they were originally invented to describe the Japanese two-fold structure of consciousness, I think this is possible because the concepts are sufficiently abstract. The fact that they refer to a very critical period of life when a child begins to distinguish between what he can say to others and what he cannot makes them particularly applicable to psychiatric thinking. For one could assume that without acquiring such a distinction a child would not come to awareness of his inner self and consequently there would be no healthy growth of his ego. Also, as I noted above, if to distinguish between *omote* and *ura* is a way of handling ambivalent feelings, it must be especially worthwhile to investigate how it fares in different psychiatric conditions.

Now what follows is a tentative sketch of my experimenting with these concepts in identifying various types of psychopathology. First, neurotics seem to be those whose *ura* threatens to come out against their better judgment. In other words, they cannot contain *ura* safely within themselves in spite of their capacity to distinguish between *omote* and *ura*. Second, psychopaths seem to be those who think they can get away with *ura*, casting *omote* to the winds. Third, epileptics seem to be those who, though ordinarily holding fast to the distinction between *omote* and *ura*, may suddenly feel compelled to discard such a distinction for a 'total' consciousness. Fourth, manic depressives seem to be those who are convinced that they have no *ura*. In other words, they have put all their heart in *omote*. But if a time comes when they can no longer maintain *omote*, *ura* will come out with all its vehemence either in the form of a manic or a depressive state. Fifth, schizophrenics seem to be those who failed to develop the sense of *omote* and *ura* at a proper developmental time. They are transparent to others and to themselves as well. So when they are later forced by external circumstances to distinguish between *omote* and *ura*, they are bound to break down into a confused state.

Thus, it seems possible to characterize various types of psychopathology in terms of *omote* and *ura*. It is simple, neat, and I believe, meaningful even without nosological nomenclature. One could perhaps say that it gives new meanings to the old nosological concepts. It has also the advantage of being able to tie up quite well with a detailed study of psychodynamics. I shall be happy indeed if this proposition is further tested by Western psychiatrists.

REFERENCES

1.   Caudill, W., and Doi, L. T. Interrelations of psychiatry, culture and emotion in Japan. In Galdston, I. Ed. *Man's Image in Medicine and Anthropology*. International Universities Press, New York, 1963.
2.   Doi, L. T. *Amae* – A key concept for understanding Japanese personality structure. In Smith, R. J., and Beardsley, R. K., Eds. *Japanese Culture: Its Development and Characteristics*. Aldine, Chicago, 1963.
3.   Doi, L. T. Giri-Ninjo: An interpretation. In Dore, R. P., Ed. *Aspects of Social Change in Modern Japan*. Princeton University Press, Princeton, New Jersey, 1967.
4.   Doi, L. T. Some thoughts on helplessness and the desire to be loved. Psychology, *26*: 266-272, 1963.
5.   James, W. *The Principles of Psychology*, vol. 1. Henry Holt and Co., New York, 1890.

First published in William P. Lebra (Ed.), *Youth Socialization and Mental Health*, East-West Center Book, University of Hawaii Press, 1974

⑭ *Higaisha-ishiki*: The Psychology of Revolting Youth in Japan

Let me introduce at the beginning *higaisha-ishiki*, the Japanese word that appears in the title. Being Japanese, I am given to using Japanese concepts, and once in a while I come upon something quite excellent which I feel like introducing to English-speaking people. *Higaisha-ishiki* is one such concept. Not that the meaning of this word cannot be rendered into English. But it happens to be handy and apt for describing a certain psychological attitude that is characteristic of the revolting youth in our contemporary world. It also has the advantage of suggesting the underlying dynamics of such an attitude,

Higaisha-ishiki is composed of two parts: *higaisha* and *ishiki*. *Higaisha*, meaning 'one who is wronged' or 'the injured party', seems to have been coined in the Meiji period as a legal term along with *kagaisha*, meaning 'one who inflicts a wrong on others' or 'perpetrator'. *Ishiki* stands for 'consciousness' and can denote 'the mentality of' when used in combination with a noun that indicates a person. Thus, *higaisha-ishiki* means 'the mentality of a person who is wronged', in other words, 'victim-consciousness'. Now *higaisha-ishiki* is quite widely used, apart from its originally legal implication, to refer to anybody who believes he has been wronged. In fact, Masao Maruyama, a well-known professor of political science at the University of Tokyo, wrote in his book *Nihon no Shisō* (*Japanese Thought*) that all Japanese, whether conservatives firmly placed within the establishment or progressives popular in communication media, tend to have *higaisha-ishiki*, a remark that I quoted in my paper on *giri-ninjō* (Doi, 1967). I shall come back to this point later.

What enlightened me on the importance of *higaisha-ishiki* as a moving force in our contemporary world was the recent student movement in Japan. Let me give a rough sketch of it. For several years, medical students fought for repeal of the law requiring internship on the ground that internship is useless and a waste of time. Their grievances were not necessarily unfounded, for postgraduate education in all fields of clinical medicine is very poor in Japan. In 1967 the medical students at the University of Tokyo, for instance, boycotted classes altogether for two months, demanding that the University Hospital provide proper training for all graduates. The professors gave in to their demands, and in the meantime the Government prepared a new law for postgraduate clinical training. In 1968 the students staged an even bigger strike, demanding a radical change in the medical education system. Their tactics became increasingly violent, and school authorities made a counterattack, taking disciplinary measures against those who menaced the hospital staff. This set the whole University on a general strike, and many young faculty members of various schools were drawn into the protest movement. At about the same time, similar upheavals swept through almost all campuses in Japan. This not only paralysed higher educational activities for more than a year, but also brought considerable damage to school buildings and facilities. Now, the campuses are much more quiet than before, but a few professional associations that sided with the universities are in trouble. For instance, the Japanese Psychiatric Association has not held its regular annual meeting since 1969. The Psychiatric Department of the University of Tokyo remains divided in two opposing camps, one centering around a certain professor, and the other, led by New Leftists, fighting to oust that professor, whom they label a sympathizer of the Japanese Communist Party.

When the foregoing incidents took place, I was amazed most of all by the speed with which the revolutionary fervor seized all the campuses. It was not only that the school authorities and the majority of students could not come up with any effective measures to put down the rioting, but a great many students and even a number of professors, though they never participated in violent activities themselves, either voiced sympathy for the rebels or publicly defended their cause. Many leading newspapers also gave the impression of being on their side by not attacking the student violence directly, though they of course duly deplored it. I found all this very appalling and strange. It was not that I felt very harsh myself toward the rebels, differently from others. On the contrary, my initial reaction was that they would not have had the chance to cause such trouble if the authorities had been more understanding and imaginative in coping with them. I guess I even identified myself with them to some extent. All the more I wondered what it is that made the adult world so helpless vis-à-vis the rebellious students.

Soon it dawned on me that the reason for our adults' helplessness was the guilt that revolting students aroused in us. Apparently they knew quite well what they were doing: they would urge those whom they had attacked, 'Don't play *higaisha* because that is only to complain, which after all is motivated by your petty egoism; convert *higaisha-ishiki* into *kagaisha-ishiki* by realizing that you yourselves have been grossly guilty of complacency in overlooking the numerous social ills.' This tactic seemed to work remarkably well. It was because of this that the rebels succeeded in recruiting many students into their camp in the first place and in silencing their critics. I wondered. then, how on earth they themselves could get away with their own guilt in the face of their almost criminal conduct, not to speak of the fact that they themselves had not done a thing to correct the social ills. This could happen, I thought, only because they completely identified themselves with the victims of the social ills, believing that they could thus negate their own privileged identity. Does it not prove, then, that they hid themselves in a sort of vicarious *higaisha-ishiki*? I think it does, only they refused to admit this to themselves. If they did, they would have had to face their own guilt by their own logic.

This identification with the supposed victims on the part of the rebellious became quite clear when a number of young radical psychiatrists began to attack the Psychiatric Association. They accused the leaders of the association of monopolizing it only to enhance their privileged positions and of neglecting to improve the conditions of mental hospitals where patients were locked in and fed large doses of tranquilizers to make them amenable to control. They also opposed a plan, which the association was then considering, to launch a system of specialty training, the rebels claiming that it was only meant to divert young physicians' attentions from social action and to keep them securely in the confines of the universities or big hospitals. Unfortunately, their accusations were not entirely un-founded. At any rate, the leaders yielded to them without much resistance and the association became totally demoralized. So we are now in a worse state than before. When all this happened I thought, it is just the reverse of the witch hunts in the European Middle Ages. Then, people projected their bad impulses onto the mentally deranged and persecuted them as witches; now, young psychiatrists project their humiliations onto the mentally deranged and completely identify themselves with the unfortu-nate. Both are the same in being paranoid. I warned them, 'If you become too involved with *higaisha*, that is, victims, you are bound to become *higaiteki*'. *Higaiteki* is an adjective often used by Japanese psychiatrists to indicate that the patient tends to have persecutory delusions. But they have not listened to my warnings.

I think it is now clear why I felt that the psychology of *higaisha-ishiki* is applicable to the youth in revolt. Of course, the phenomenon of dissident youth is not confined to Japan alone; on the contrary, it is spread throughout the contemporary world. Almost identical student riots occurred at Berkeley, Harvard, in Paris, and many other places. As a matter of fact, I have often been struck by the similarity of the ideology and tactics used by youth in various countries. It followed that the psychology of *higaisha-ishiki* might also be applicable to the revolting youth in other countries besides Japan. This thought intrigued me because the psychology of *higaisha-ishiki* as I formulated it above is clearly a derivative of the psychology of *amae*, that is, the particular dependency need that manifests itself in a longing to merge with others in a loving relationship. Those who are totally engrossed in *amae* would develop *higaisha-ishiki* when they feel rejected. It is easy to understand, therefore, that the Japanese people tend to have, *higaisha-ishiki*, as Professor Maruyama pointed out. One might even hazard the thesis that what motivated Japan to wage her last war against the United States is also related to this psychology. Justly or unjustly, Japan felt persecuted by the United States and started on a war which she did not believe she could win. She may have hoped that the United States would feel guilty afterwards; if so she was quite right. Because Americans had to feel terribly guilty, particularly after dropping the atomic bombs, the initial victim of Japan's surprise attack was made to feel like the guilty one in the end. In the words made popular by the recent Japanese student riots, in this instance *higaisha-ishiki* was more or less successfully converted into *kagaisha-ishiki*.

So there is a distinct parallel between the *higaisha-ishiki* of contemporary Japanese youth against the establishment and that of their fathers against the United States or other powerful foreign countries. But why against the establishment at the present time? Also, how does one explain the fact that now youth in Western countries are also caught by *higaisha-ishiki*? It is interesting to note in this regard that it is the threat of nuclear holocaust that now prevents the conflicts between powerful nations from escalating into hot war, thus creating the precarious cold peace and leading to the revolt of youth against the established authorities in advanced countries. For a long time, the West enjoyed the aggressor role on the world stage because of its advancement in science and technology. But now, that very advancement has created new problems for the West such as environmental pollution. The West's liberation of its former colonies in the present century also owes to social changes created by the advanced technology. Thus, conditions became ripe for the youth in Western countries to develop *higaisha-ishiki*, either by anticipating the possible dead end of contemporary civilization or by identification with the underprivileged. It is significant that Erik H. Erikson (1970) calls the present youth unrest 'revolt of the dependent', not 'revolt of the oppressed'. He must mean the same thing I mean by *higaisha-ishiki*.

I would like to add a few more words about the connection between *higaisha-ishiki* and paranoid thinking that I hinted at above. I think the usual psychiatric conception of persecutory delusions is that they represent projections of the patient's own hostile feelings onto the external object. This is quite right, but I wonder if Western people do not sometimes forget that the hostility is originally engendered by frustration of one's deep dependency wishes, that is, *amae* in Japanese. Though some psychiatrists in the West recently pointed out a connection between an initial traumatic experience and later paranoid development, they did so only in extreme cases like the Nazi survivors. Robert J. Lifton (1967) came to a similar conclusion by observing the acute suspicion of 'counterfeit nurture' among the atomic bomb survivors of Hiroshima. Apart from these striking examples, however, it is my impression that Western people tend to overlook the paranoid reaction that is provoked by the frustration of dependency wishes, particularly when it is mild. This applies, surprisingly, even to a psychological genius like Freud.

Let me cite, for instance, from 'Analysis of a Phobia in a Five-Year-Old Boy', a passing conversation between Hans and his father, who actually took the role of therapist for Hans through the help of Freud (1950). His father asks him, 'What do I really scold you for?' He answers, 'I don't know.' His father presses, 'Why?', to which he says, 'Because you're cross.' His father denies it, saying, 'But that's not true,' but Hans emphatically repeats, 'Yes, it is true. You're cross. I know you are. It must be true.' His father then notes the following. 'Evidently, therefore, my explanation that only little boys come into bed with their Mummies and that big ones sleep in their own beds had not impressed him very much.' Now one could have said that Hans projected his hostile feelings onto his father. But was he not right after all in insisting that his father was cross? (In the original German, 'You are cross' is *Du tust eifern*.) The father's flat denial of this charge rather makes one suspect that it was perhaps the father who projected his anger toward Hans, which was caused by his wife allowing Hans to sleep with her. The fact that this marriage eventually ended in divorce strongly supports this interpretation. However, Freud takes notice neither of such a paranoid feeling on the part of Hans' father nor of the possibility that the father's mute anger or the couple's incompatibility might have been a main contributing factor for Hans' phobic neurosis.

Interestingly, it seems that Freud himself experienced such a paranoid feeling at times without recognizing it as such. I shall cite one example. In *The Interpretation of Dreams* (1961), he faithfully recorded his reaction to what he heard from his colleague Otto about the condition of his patient Irma, whom he had treated only with partial success. 'I asked him how he had found her and he answered: "She's better, but not quite well." I was conscious that my friend Otto's words, or the tone in which he spoke them, annoyed me. I fancied I detected a reproof in them, such as to the effect that I had promised the patient too much; and, whether rightly or wrongly, I attributed the supposed fact of Otto's siding against me to the influence of my patient's relatives, who, as it seemed to me, had never looked with favour on the treatment.' Is it not quite clear that Freud was slightly paranoid here? It may be true that Irma's family did not feel kindly toward Freud's novel treatment and that Otto was not particularly sympathetic to it either. Even if so, Freud had no reason to blame them. On the other hand, it is most certain that the treatment of Irma had left him unsatisfied and that is why he was so unduly sensitive to Otto's report about her. It can be said, therefore, that the famous Irma dream was actually a continuation of this paranoid reaction, but curiously so far no analyst has come up with such an impious interpretation.

It is my contention that this kind of paranoid reaction is widespread in the contemporary world. The examples I gave above are mild ones, but such a reaction can be quite destructive when it takes a mass form, as in the case of revolting youth. Unfortunately, nobody has paid much attention to the psychological aspect of rebellious youth; such a phenomenon is usually analyzed only in sociological or political terms. Recently, however, Stuart Hughes, a distinguished Harvard professor of history, mentioned the present youth revolt in his special address to the 1969 annual meeting of the American Psychiatric Association:

> What has been unusual about the insurgent mood of the past half decade has been its juxtaposition of anarchism and the peremptory silencing of opponents, its peculiar blend of political puritanism and personal license, its cult of 'confrontation' as a quasi-religious act of witness. Together this complex of attitudes suggests something quite different from the conventional revolutionary aim of seizing the means of production or the implements of power and redirecting them for the benefit of the masses. It suggests, rather, a basically unpolitical aspiration to see through, to unmask, to strip – literally as well as figuratively – down to total nakedness. The goal is psychological, or, to use old-fashioned vocabulary, spiritual. And it marks the culmination of a quarter-century of amateur psychologizing among the young. (Hughes, 1969)

Evidently he was keenly aware of the psychological aspect of the present youth revolt, but I don't know of any American psychiatrist who sufficiently clarified the issue for him.

In this connection I would like to mention *Contestation*, a brilliant study of the Paris student revolt of May, 1968, by two eminent French psychoanalysts, B. Brunberger and J.S. Smirgel (1969). It makes amply clear the paranoid nature of what motivated those youth who contested the authorities, and is in complete agreement with my own view of Japanese youth. But their emphasis is again on the projection of hostility. Though they noticed the youth's identification with the supposed victims of society, they did so only in a tone of ridicule. They thus stopped short of recognizing the importance of frustrated dependency wishes in forming the paranoid reaction. In other words, the authors are not perceptive to the feelings of humiliation that must have existed deep down in the hearts of those youth who revolted. In my opinion, Western people generally, youth and professional adults alike, have not been attentive to such feelings of humiliation and do not dwell on them, either by repressing or suppressing them.

I am aware that I have put forward a very sweeping generalization. I did so not because I wanted to indulge in speculation, but because I felt it has a practical clinical merit. I only wanted to tell you that many young people who consult psychiatrists nowadays have the kind of paranoid reaction explained above, in other words, *higaisha-ishiki*, if not in a mass form, then as a solitary preoccupation. I conclude with a plea that psychiatrists, Japanese and non-Japanese alike, work to gain insight into this psychology and what lies behind it, that is, the particular dependency need called *amae*.

REFERENCES

Brunberger. B., and J.S. Smirgel. 1969. *Contestation*. Paris. Payot. [In French]
Doi, L.T. 1967. *Giri-ninjo*: an interpretation. In *Aspects of social change in modern Japan*. R.P. Dore, ed. Princeton, Princeton University Press.
Erikson, E.H. 1970. Reflections on the dissent of contemporary youth. *International Journal of Psychoanalysis* 51: 11-22.
Freud, S. 1950. Analysis of a phobia in a five-year-old boy. *Collected papers*. Vol. 3. London, The Hogarth Press.
—— 1961. *The interpretation of dreams*. New York, Science Editions, Inc.
Hughes, E.S. 1969. Emotional disturbance and American social change, 1944-1969. *American Journal of Psychiatry* 126:21-29.
Lifton, R.J. 1967. *Death in life*. New York, Random House.

First published in Albert M. Craig (Ed.), *Japan: A Comparative View*. © Princeton University Press, 1979

⑮ Uchimura Kanzō: Japanese Christianity in Comparative Perspective

This chapter is a study of Uchimura Kanzō (1861-1930), particularly his personality development and its bearing on his Christian beliefs. My objective is to define the distinctly Japanese quality of his Christianity as compared with that of non-Japanese Christians. Uchimura himself was a prolific writer, and there are numerous articles and books on his life and work, but for my purposes I shall focus mainly on the book he wrote in English, *How I Became a Christian*.[1]

Uchimura was one of the few pioneers in offering his own experiences as a Japanese for the benefit of non-Japanese. He began writing *How I Became a Christian* in 1893 and wanted to have it published in the United States. However, after the manuscript's initial rejection by an American publisher, it was published in Japan in 1895, followed by the American edition which appeared later the same year under the title *The Diary of a Japanese Convert*. In the preface to the Japanese edition, Uchimura wrote as follows:

> In many a religious gathering, to which I was invited during my stay in America to give a talk for fifteen minutes and no more (as some great doctor, the chief speaker of the meeting, was to fill up most of the time), I often asked the chairman (or the chairwoman) what they would like to hear from me. The commonest answer I received was, 'Oh, just tell us how you were converted.' I was always at a loss how to comply with such a demand, as I could not in any way tell in 'fifteen minutes and no more' the awful change that came over my soul since I was brought in contact with Christianity. The fact is, the conversion of a heathen is always a matter of wonder, if not of curiosity, to the Christian public; and it was just natural that I too was asked to tell them some vivid accounts of how 'I threw my idols into the fire, and clung unto the Gospel'. (p. 9).

One can hardly miss the hidden irony in the preceding passage, indicating a protest against what Uchimura thought to be the patronizing attitude on the part of American Christians. It was evidently to redress such an attitude and make them view his experience of conversion more seriously that he wrote *How I Became a Christian*. Of course, affront was not the sole motivation for writing this book. Uchimura was thirty-three when he began writing it, five years after his return from the United States and still several years before settling on his life-work. It is likely that he wanted to review his

97

experiences for himself, so that he could better face whatever would be in store for him in the coming years. In other words, the book constituted for him an attempt to consolidate his identity. The following words in his introduction to the book suggest such a view:

> I early contracted the habit of keeping my diary, in which I noted down whatever ideas and events that came to pass upon me. I made myself a subject of careful observation, and found it more mysterious than anything I ever have studied. I jotted down its rise and progress, its falls and backslidings, its joys and hopes, its sins and darkness; and notwithstanding all the awfulness that attends such an observation like this, I found it more seriously interesting than any study I ever have undertaken. (p. 15).

It is remarkable that Uchimura found self-observation so interesting, but perhaps even more remarkable that he thought his observations would be interesting to the public as well. What was offered the public could not be exactly what he jotted down in his diary. He certainly edited the material, and it is known that he discreetly withheld any concrete information about his first marriage. Also, he destroyed the diary after completion of the book. Perhaps he reasoned that the book was a distillation of his past experiences, the only thing of value that could be presented to the public.

Valuable in what sense? Uchimura does not specify, leaving that judgment up to the reader by saying, 'The reader may draw whatever conclusions he likes from it' (p. 15). Still he was convinced that the book had a message for the wider public and even hoped that it would sell well in the United States. He was disappointed when its sales did not go as well as he had wished. It is reported that the first edition of five hundred copies took several years to be sold, and that the book then went out of print. Against this background one can imagine his pleasant surprise when the German version was published in 1904, and three thousand copies sold at once. He deduced from this that German readers had a better understanding of what he had to say because they were heirs to Martin Luther's Christianity. But, perhaps more significantly, the publication of the German version coincided with the outbreak of the Russo-Japanese War, which certainly aroused worldwide interest in Japan and the Japanese.

In what follows I shall first analyze the contents of the book and compare it with Erik Erikson's analysis of Luther's formative years.[2] I shall then discuss Uchimura's later life from the vantage point provided by this analysis. Finally, I shall attempt to clarify his position by comparison with several Christian thinkers in the West and to summarize the features that characterize his brand of Christianity as uniquely Japanese.

THE FORMATIVE YEARS

In the beginning of the first chapter of the book, entitled 'Heathenism', Uchimura gives a brief sketch of his family background. On first reading it, one gets little information about what kind of relationship he had with his parents, except that in describing them he is dutifully filial and treats them with care, affection, and reverence. But if one tries to read between the lines, one glimpses what might actually have transpired between him and his parents. I shall first take up the father-son relationship.

He introduces his father as follows: 'My father was cultured, could write good poetry, and was learned in the art of ruling men. He too was a man of no mean military ability, and could lead a most turbulent regiment in a very creditable way' (p. 17). This description clearly indicates the son's pride in his father, but in the following paragraph he reports a curious episode, which apparently taxed his nerves sorely. 'My father was decidedly blasphemous toward heathen gods of all sorts. He once dropped a base coin into the money-chest of a Buddhist temple, and scornfully addressed the idols that they would have another such coin if they would in anyway help him to win a law-case in which he was then engaged; a feat wholly beyond my power at any period of my religious experience' (pp. 18-19). This passage comes right after the statement, 'But to no one of them do I trace the origin of my "religious sensibilities", which I early acquired in my boyhood' (p. 18).

So it appears that Uchimura became religious in spite of his father. As a young boy he surely could not have accused his father of blasphemy. But the first thing he did when he was later converted to Christianity was vigorously to attempt to convert his father. His first attempt, which took place when he returned home from college for vacation, was not successful. He states that 'my mother was indifferent, my father was decidedly antagonistic, and my younger brother. . . was so provoking. . .' (p. 47). However, he must have pressed his father hard, because finally he says, 'I succeeded in extracting from my father a promise to examine the faith I implored him to receive' (p. 48). His second attempt at winning over his father, which came two years later, was successful. The idea suddenly occurred to him of giving his father the *Commentary on the Gospel of St. Mark* consisting of five volumes, written by Dr. Faber, a German missionary in China. Why he did it and how it was received by his father is described as follows.

> It [the *Commentary*] was written in unpointed Chinese, and I thought the difficulty of reading it, if not anything else, might whet my father's intellectual appetite to pursue it. I invested two dollars upon this work, and carried it in my trunk to my father. But alas! When I gave it to my father, no words of thanks or appreciation came from his lips, and all the best wishes of my heart met his coldest reception. I went into a closet and wept. The books were throw into a box with other rubbish; but I took out the first volume and left it on his table. In his leisure when he had nothing else to do, he would read a page or so, and again it went into the rubbish. I took it out again, and placed it on his table as before. My patience was as great as his reluctance to read these books. Finally, however, I prevailed; he went through the first volume! He stopped scoffing at Christianity! Something in the book must have touched his heart! I did the same thing with the second volume as with the first. Yes, he finished the second volume too, and he began to speak favorably of Christianity. Thank God, he was coming. He finished the third volume, and I observed some change in his life and

manners. He would drink less wine, and his behavior toward his wife and children was becoming more affectionate than before. The fourth volume was finished, and his heart came down! 'Son,' he said, 'I have been a poor man. From this day, you may be sure, I will be a disciple of Jesus.' I took him to a church, and observed in him the convulsion of his whole nature. Everything he heard there moved him. The eyes that were all masculine and soldierly were now wet with tears. He would not touch his wine any more. Twelve months more and he was baptized. (p. 72).

The son had used a clever trick, and it worked. Even though the battle was fierce, the son finally prevailed over the father. However, this is not to suggest that Uchimura had no genuine respect and affection for his father. It suggests only that he could not look to him for spiritual guidance. Perhaps his father never meant much as an authority figure for him, and that is why he presented himself as a new authority to his father. Father and son had exchanged their customary roles, and it was as if the son were trying to teach the wayward father without being disgusted by him. It was fortunate for the father that Kanzō succeeded in this audacious enterprise, for he could from then on count on his father's moral support.

That such was the nature of Uchimura's relationship to his father is supported by information from other sources. Uchimura was made the head of the whole household when he entered Sapporo Agricultural College at sixteen, as his father had retired a few years before in his early forties. This meant that besides his parents, Uchimura had three younger brothers and one younger sister to look after. All this gives credence to the story that he volunteered to go to Sapporo Agricultural College – situated in Hokkaido, still undeveloped and far removed to the north from the capital – only because there he could receive free tuition, plus room and board, with a handsome stipend from which he could contribute to the upkeep of his family. From that time Uchimura and his father switched their respective roles.

Concerning his relationship with his mother Uchimura has this to say: 'My mother has inherited from her mother this mania for work. She forgets all the pain and sorrow of life in her work. She is one of those who can't afford to be gloomy because life is hard. Her little home is her kingdom, and she rules it, washes it, feeds it, as no queen has ever done' (p. 18). In this thumbnail sketch of Uchimura's mother, what strikes me most is his use of the word *mania* (he italicized it). It is a strong word and can even be slightly pejorative. Prior to describing his mother, he affectionately describes his maternal grandmother as a lovable old lady. She had been a widow for fifty years and had reared all five children by herself – she was a hard worker by necessity. In comparison with this grandmother, however, one gets the impression that Uchimura's mother was a hard worker by compulsion, even though, as he says, she somehow 'inherited from her mother this mania for work'. She is presented as single-minded, indomitable, and perhaps even inaccessible. She appears twice at a later stage in the book, and again she gives the same impression as the earlier one.

I have already mentioned that his mother was indifferent when Uchimura first tried to convert his family to Christianity. He states, 'I told my mother that I became a new man in Sapporo, and that she too must become what I became. But she was so much taken up with the joy of seeing her son again that she cared nothing about what I told her about Christianity' (p. 47). Toward the end of the book, where the family reunion after his three-and-a-half-year stay in America is described, he again states that 'Mother doesn't care to learn about the world; she is only glad that her son is safely at home', whereas he 'talked with father all night' (p. 209).

What kind of mother does not care to listen to what her beloved son wants to tell her? Was she cold? She must have loved him in her own way. But she was only glad to have him back and could not appreciate his experience of growing up in the world. Was she possibly too possessive? Could her attitude have hurt the sensitive Uchimura? He does not say, but instead, right after the briefly quoted description, he relates once more the scene of his homecoming: '"Mama", I cried as I opened the gate, "your son is back again." Her lean form, with many more marks of toil upon it, how beautiful! The ideal beauty that I failed to recognize in the choices of my Delaware friend, I found again in the sacred form of my mother' (p. 210). This unmistakably suggests a case of idealization of his mother.

From all this I conclude that Uchimura was not close to his mother, much as he might have wished to be. At least he was close to his father. Still, as I suggested before, he could not really depend on his father either. In terms of *amae*, one could say that he did not *amaeru* as a child toward his parents. Perhaps this was partially because as the oldest of five children from an early age he felt keenly the responsibility for the household. Did the frustration in *amae* affect his personality? I think his early religiosity, which I discuss in the next section, is definitely related to this. Also, his reason for attempting to convert his parents to 'become what I became' bespeaks his strong sense of being bound to them. He could easily have left them behind and alone. This, however, he did not do. Instead it was as though he had to bind them, precisely because he was bound to them by a hidden need. I think this clearly indicates his frustrated *amae*, a desperate attempt to capture the never freely given affection of his parents.

That Uchimura was particularly sensitive to the feeling of *amae* is shown by his emphatic use of the mother symbol throughout the book.[3] He describes the moment of separation when he left Japan for America in the following words:

> Love of country, like all other loves, is at its best and highest at the time of separation. That strange Something, which, when at home, is no more to us than a mere grouping of rills and valleys, mountains and hills, is now transformed to that living Somebody – Nature etherealized into a spirit – and as a woman speaks to her children, it summons us to noble deeds. . . .
> The yonder imperial peak that hangs majestically against the western snow – is that not her chaste brow, the inspirer of the nation's heart? The pine-clad

hills that encircle the peak, and golden fields that in its bottom lie – is that not the bosom that suckled me, and the knee that took me up? A mother so pure, so noble and lovely – shall not her sons be loyal to her? (pp. 103-104).

Again, in reminiscing of his college days at Amherst College, he states, 'I am exceedingly thankful that I was given another such mother to serve and satisfy' (p. 167). And, there is a passage in which he refers to the Spirit of God as 'my Mama' (p. 154). I do not know of any Western Christian who specifically used the mother symbol for the Holy Spirit of the Trinity. From all this one could conclude that Uchimura was always looking for the mother figure who would satisfy his *amae*, as his own parents, particularly his mother, did not.[4]

□

Let me now turn to Martin Luther's relationship with his parents. He was the first son of Hans Luder, an ambitious ex-peasant who engaged in mining, a new industry in Germany at that time. Hans wanted his son to become a lawyer, and Martin dutifully obeyed the father's wish up to the age of twenty-one, when suddenly, following the famous thunderstorm experience, he quit the study of law he had just begun at the University of Erfurt and entered an Augustinian monastery. Hans was furious and would not give his consent or fatherly blessing. Apparently his wife followed suit. This incident clearly shows that Luther's relationship with his father was quite different from Kanzō's, and it weighed much more for him than his relationship with his mother. Luther's father would not relinquish his hold on the son easily, and perhaps he never did. It is interesting to note in this respect that when Luther, having broken with the Church, was married, he stated as his first and foremost reason that it would please his father.[5] Luther made two remarks in later life about his parents: 'My father once whipped me so that *I fled him and became sadly resentful toward him, until he gradually got me accustomed to him again*'; '*My mother caned me for stealing a nut and afterwards there was blood. Such strict discipline drove me into monkery or the monk-business.*'[6] (The italicized portions are Erikson's literal translation from German.) Erikson concludes:

> Martin, even when mortally afraid, could not really hate his father, he could only be sad; and Hans, while he could not let the boy come close, and was murderously angry at times, could not let him go for long. They had a mutual and deep investment in each other which neither of them could or would abandon, although neither of them was able to bring it to any kind of fruition. . . . The monk-business refers to his [Luther's] exaggeration of the ascetic and the scrupulous. He implies strongly, then, that such treatment was responsible for the excessive, the neurotic side of the religionism of his early twenties.[7]

About this neurotic side of Luther more will be said in comparison with Uchimura's religious development.

EARLY RELIGIOSITY

I have already mentioned Uchimura's 'religious sensibilities', which he says he acquired early in his boyhood. Here I shall quote his description of how excessively religious he was, long before he was converted to Christianity:

> I believed, and that sincerely, that there dwelt in each of innumerable temples its god, jealous over its jurisdiction, ready with punishment to any transgressor that fell under his displeasure. The god whom I reverenced and adored most was the god of learning and writing, for whom I faithfully observed the 25th of every month with due sanctity and sacrifice. I prostrated myself before his image, earnestly implored his aid to improve my hand-writing and help my memory. Then there is a god who presides over rice-culture, and his errands unto mortals are white foxes. He can be approached with prayers to protect our houses from fire and robbery, and as my father was mostly away from the house, and I was alone with my mother, I ceased not to beseech this god of rice to keep my poor house from the said disasters. There was another god whom I feared more than all others. His emblem was a black raven, and he was the searcher of man's inmost heart. The keeper of his temple issued papers upon which ravens were printed in sombre colors, the whole having a miraculous power to cause immediate haemorrhage when taken into stomach by any one who told falsehood. I often vindicated my truthfulness before my comrades by calling upon them to test my veracity by the use of a piece of this sacred paper, if they stood in suspicion of what I asserted. Still another god exercised healing power upon those who suffer from toothache. Him also did I call upon, as I was a constant sufferer from this painful malady. He would exact from his devotee a vow to abstain from pears as specially obnoxious to him. . . . One god would impose upon me abstinence from the use of eggs, another from beans, till after I made all my vows, many of my boyish delicacies were entered upon the prohibition list. Multiplicity of gods often involved the contradiction of the requirements of one god with those of another, and sad was the plight of a conscientious soul when he had to satisfy more than one god. With so many gods to satisfy and appease, I was naturally a fretful, timid child, I framed a general prayer to be offered to every one of them, adding of course special requests appropriate to each, as I happened to pass before each temple. . . . Where several temples were contiguous to one another, the trouble of repeating the same prayer so many times was very great; and I would often prefer a longer route with less number of sanctuaries in order to avoid the trouble of saying my prayers without scruples of conscience. The number of deities to be worshipped increased day by day, till I found my little soul totally incapable of pleasing them all (p. 23).

The picture given here is certainly that of a precocious boy who is pitiably scrupulous in offering correct worship to each of the numerous gods. Uchimura prefaces the preceding description with the sentence, 'But no retrospect of my bygone days causes in me a greater humiliation than the spiritual darkness I groped under, laboriously sustained with gross superstitions' (pp. 21-22). Very few, if any, however, would dare to laugh at him for his so sincere 'superstitions'. Surely his scrupulosity would fall into the neurotic range. But what is important is not to label him as obsessive-compulsive, but to understand the underlying anxiety which is so palpable. And speaking of anxiety, he writes later in the book that he used to be afraid of thunder, saying, 'I always thought my end did come when it rattled right above my head. In my heathen days, I called in the help of all my protecting gods, burnt incense to them, and took my refuge under a mosquito-net as the safest place to flee from "the wrath of heaven"' (p. 156). It seems certain that his religiosity was closely tied up with his proneness to anxiety and perhaps could be interpreted as a means of coping with it.

The question to be asked, then, is why Uchimura was given to so much anxiety. By this I do not mean to say that religion is simply a function of anxiety. Again, given his anxiety, why it took the form of 'religious sensibilities' is another question which does not concern me at the moment. To get back to the question I originally posed, it is significant that the sentence in which he disavowed any influence from his relatives on his 'religious sensibilities' was inserted between the mention of his mother and his father. It is a clinical axiom that if and when a patient tells logically disconnected things together, one can assume the existence of an emotional connection between them. I think this axiom can apply to the case of Uchimura. In other words, I want to propose here that his early religiosity was definitely linked to his parents, notwithstanding his claim that its origin cannot be traced to either of them.

To make the preceding proposition more plausible, I shall relate here something about the background of the Uchimura family. They were *samurai* in one of the pro-Tokugawa domains; the overthrow of the Tokugawa government then led them to personal disaster. This would explain at least partially Kanzō's father's much too early retirement; he must have felt at odds with the revolutionary changes around him. In this connection I also wonder if the recorded blasphemy of Uchimura's father was not more expressive of his anger against the fate that had befallen him rather than against a Buddha. We can be sure at least that he did not inspire the strength and confidence in the members of his family that he should have. Read once more the following passage in the preceding quotation: '. . . as my father was mostly away from home, and I was alone with my mother, I ceased not to beseech this god of rice to keep my poor home from the said disasters' (p. 22). That Uchimura felt helplessness and anxiety in the company of his mother sounds pathetic. It almost reads as if, to the great distress of his mother, his father had deserted the family although presumably he was kept away from home because of work. Or could it be that Uchimura instinctively sensed the hidden anxiety of his mother, which in turn made him so anxious? In this context the word *mania* which he used to describe the way his mother worked acquires a new implication, for was not his way of worshipping gods also mania-like? He went around worshipping gods to ward off his own misgivings, just as his mother has 'this mania of work' to forestall any misfortune. There can be no denying a definite resemblance between the two, whether an inherited or infected one.

I would like to make one last comment on Uchimura's early religiosity, particularly with regard to the cult of a god who 'was the searcher of man's inmost heart'. He says he feared this god more than all others and would often swear his truthfulness by the god's miraculous power. It shows his fine moral sensibility, which in itself should be lauded. But if one asks whether he swore often because he feared the god, the answer must be the converse. The more he swore, the more he must have feared the god. Such is the dilemma of moral scrupulosity. Uchimura's ambivalence had gotten out of hand. In other words, he somehow could not get used to the Japanese custom of solving ambivalence by alternately playing *omote* and *ura* and therefore was more vulnerable to any personal affront. So he swore often, and, swearing, he feared even more the god who was searching his heart. He did not find a way out of this dilemma for quite some time even after Christianity came to his rescue.[8]

Compared with Uchimura's early religiosity, which stands out against the unreligious stance of his parents, Martin Luther's seems to stem directly from his parents, who never questioned the medieval religious *Weltanschauung* and its many superstitions. Only their harshness in disciplining him must have made him overly docile and scrupulous, as was suggested in his remarks quoted in the previous section. Thus Martin became a sad young man full of conflicts, and it was because of those conflicts that he quit his studies and entered a monastery against his father's ardent wish. It is interesting that in the very act of disobeying his father he called upon St. Anne, the patron saint of his father's trade, for help. Stricken with fear in a thunderstorm, he called out, 'Help me, St. Anne . . . I want to become a monk.'[9] As Erikson suggests, he probably wanted her to intercede with his father in the confrontation that must follow.

Be that as it may, it is certain that in his decision to enter the monastery Martin was beset with ambivalent feelings toward his father, who had decided on a worldly career for him. Two years later, when he celebrated his first mass, he asked his father, who had been invited as a guest, 'Dear father, why did you resist so hard and become so angry because you did not want to let me be a monk, and maybe even now you do not like too much to see me here, although it is a sweet and godly life, full of peace?'[10] He was obviously trying to appease his father at this last moment, but his father retorted in front of the entire congregation, 'You scholars, have you not read in the scriptures that one should honor father and mother?'[11] Martin must have cited the thunderstorm experience and argued that his vocation was clearly from God. But his father is reported to have cried out what amounted to a curse: 'God give that it wasn't a devil's spook!'[12] Thus Luther's confrontation with his father did not end in an easy victory, as in the case of Uchimura.

FIRST CONTACT WITH CHRISTIANITY

Christianity did not come to Uchimura by inner persuasion. It came rather by force. In Tokyo, he had been introduced to churchgoing by a friend. He enjoyed the exotic sights and sounds of Christian worship but did not take it seriously. When he entered Sapporo Agricultural College, he had no idea he was going into the midst of a totally Christian-spirited group, who were prepared to catch him as if he were a prey. He found himself, along with other classmates, surrounded by upperclassmen who exerted strong pressure on newcomers to sign the 'Covenant of Believers in Jesus', a pledge which William S. Clark had penned for his students. Clark had left by then, but his influence was still evident in the zeal he had inspired in his students. Uchimura withstood their pressure for a few months, even after a number of his classmates had signed the covenant, but finally he too signed it although his inner doubts were not completely dispelled. Of this act he relates, 'The public opinion of the college was too strong against me, it was beyond my power to withstand. So, you see, my first step toward Christianity was a forced one, against my will, and I must confess, somewhat against my conscience too' (p. 26).

From this one should not surmise that Uchimura was simply coerced into accepting Christianity. He had been susceptible from the very beginning. He states, 'The practical advantage of the new faith was evident to me at once. I had felt it even while I was engaging all my powers to repel it from me' (p. 28). The advantage lay in the fact that he now had only one god to worship, whereas before he had agonized over meeting mutually conflicting demands of various gods. After his fateful decision he experienced a new exhilaration of the spirit as well as freedom of his body, as he was no longer hampered by any of his former religious scruples. So he says, 'I was not sorry that I was forced to sign the covenant' (p. 29). It is interesting to note here that it was none other than his early religiosity which made him both rejective of and receptive toward Christianity. He confesses later on, 'Indeed, the first and greatest fear I had when I was first induced to accept Christianity was that they might make a priest out of me' (p. 171) – an uncanny premonition of what he eventually became! Still, for all the attractions Christianity held for him, it was also true that he had bowed his head to a foreign god in order to take the line of least resistance against group pressure. Thus his first contact with Christianity was both liberating and traumatic. One could say that in a sense he never completely recovered from this trauma.

After signing the covenant he became an active member of the group which met every Sunday for prayer and Bible study. Several months later he was baptized along with six others in his class by M. C. Harris, an American Methodist missionary. He then adopted *Jonathan* as his Christian name because, he says, he 'was a strong advocate of the virtue of friendship' (p. 32). In fact he made lifelong friends among this group and enjoyed their company as much in social gatherings or excursions as in religious activities. They always had their own Sunday services, with each of them taking the role of pastor in turn. He records with obvious relish the excitement they shared as well as some squabbles and mischief which they unexpectedly fell into while holding services. Soon they came to realize, however, that Christianity had its own difficulties. What particularly pained them was the fact that they were divided by denomination, whether Methodist or Episcopalian. They came to grips with this problem right after graduation of the upperclassmen, perhaps because they realized that from then on those who belonged to different denominations would seldom have a chance to meet. Uchimura expresses this sentiment thus: '"Men who ate rice out of the same kettle" is our popular saying about the intimacy well nigh approaching the bond of blood-relationship; and we believed and still believe in the necessity of some other bonds of union for those who are to fight and suffer for one and the same cause than the breaking of bread and drinking of wine by the hand of an officiating minister. Could such a bond be divided into "two churches" even though ministers of two different denominations wrote the sign of the Cross upon our foreheads?' (p. 58).

They thereupon decided to build a church of their own and a committee of five members including Uchimura was elected. The news of an offer of four hundred dollars by a representative of the Methodist Episcopal Church of America encouraged them, although they did not want to accept it as a gift, but rather decided to borrow it. They clearly wanted to have an independent church with no strings attached. It seems that Kanzō was a leading spirit behind this bold enterprise, as he was, in his own words, 'young, idealistic, and impulsive and 'would pour out his heart' whenever he spoke (pp. 64 and 39). After graduation he plunged vigorously into their joint task while conducting fishery surveys as a governmental official to earn a living. Finally a half of one building was procured, and the desire to unite brethren belonging to separate denominations into one independent church was fulfilled. It was a completely lay church, and as in school days some of the members who were recent graduates from the college took turns preaching. Only one problem remained, that of paying their debt, which suddenly became urgent, for the donor requested to be paid back, as he could not approve of their independent church. It was a stupendous feat that they could pay back everything in less than two years, even though they received an unexpected gift of one hundred dollars from Clark, then in America. All of the congregation were still young and barely managing to make ends meet.

What interests me most about their enterprise is not that they succeeded in building an independent church which was completely lay in organization. Neither is it the budding ecumenism, in itself quite striking considering that it has come to see its day only recently the world over. It is rather what inspired them to launch such an enterprise. I have mentioned their initial motivation, and Uchimura further elaborated on this:

> They do err who think that our church-independence was intended as an open rebellion against the denomination to which we once belonged. It

was a humble attempt to reach the one great aim we had in view, namely, to come to the full consciousness of our own powers and capabilities, and to remove obstacles in the way of others seeking God's truth for the salvation of their souls (p. 87).

In short, he attests that what he embarked upon with others was not a protest against the established order. But in actuality it was such. Would it be too farfetched to think Uchimura took revenge for having been forced to bow his head to a foreign god by building an independent church free of foreign influences? Or perhaps this was an attempt to maintain the esprit de corps, which had been such a menace to the lonely Uchimura at the beginning, but later on came to sustain him so much in the name of Christianity. I shall come back to a discussion of this question in connection with his later pronouncement of *Mukyōkai* (Non-church), for I believe it was inspired by a similar spirit. We shall see that in both instances he defends his position in much the same way.

A VACUUM IN THE HEART

Uchimura left Sapporo for Tokyo in December 1882, apparently in a most dejected state of mind. In the chapter which describes this period of his life in Tokyo, he first introduces a quotation from Hosea (2:14-16), a prophet of the Old Testament, which are the words of God addressing stray Israel to lure her into the wilderness where He may let her recall her first fidelity. He goes on to say:

> So my Lord and Husband must have said to Himself when He drove me from my peaceful home-church. He did this by creating a vacuum in my heart. Nobody goes to a desert who has his all in his home. Nature abhors a vacuum, and the human heart abhors it more than anything else in the Universe. I descried in myself an empty space which neither activity in religious works, nor success in scientific experiments, could fill. What the exact nature of that emptiness was, I was not able to discern. Maybe my health was getting poor, and I yearned after repose and easier tasks. Or, as I was rapidly growing into my manhood, that irresistible call of nature for companionship might have made me feel so haggard and empty. At all events, a vacuum there was, something there was in this vague universe which could make me feel happy and contented; but I had no idea whatever of what that something was. Like a pigeon that was deprived of its cerebrum by the knife of a physiologist, I started, not knowing whither and wherefore, but because stay I could not. From this time on, my whole energy was thrown into this one task of filling up this vacuum (pp. 90-91).

This passage clearly indicates an acute sense of disillusionment which was instrumental in driving him from Sapporo to Tokyo. But why disillusionment? Was he not happily and proudly working for his church? He wrote in his diary on December 28, 1882, the day he completed the last payment of debt for his church, 'Joys inexpressible and indescribable!' (p. 86.) Does this note of joy contradict the preceding passage? It may be that he did not wish to acknowledge the sense of disillusionment which had been plaguing him for some time until he had completed his last duty. Still, why disillusionment? One plausible answer is that he was thoroughly disgusted with what he saw at his job, namely, the corruption among governmental officials in Hokkaido, and thought of resigning his position when he went to Tokyo, which he actually did a few months later. Strangely, he does not mention this, but instead gives a definite impression that his distress was much deeper and that he himself did not understand what could have caused it.

His condition at that time was probably what would have been diagnosed by a clinician as depression. And if I may conjecture further, I should say that his case was rather close to what Freud described as 'those wrecked by success',[13] for so far he had been enormously successful in many ways. He had graduated from college at the top of his class and was launched on a promising career, already having made a scientific discovery in his field. He had converted his antagonistic father and built, against the wishes of foreign missionaries, the only independent church then in Japan. Surely to accomplish all this he must have worked extremely hard, and he was very likely worn out. But if it was a matter of exhaustion, he could easily have recovered, for he was then only twenty-two years old. The cause of his depression must be sought somewhere deep in his mind. It is quite possible that he somehow felt guilty for his accomplishments, as Freud postulated for 'those wrecked by success'. And, with or without guilt he might have been feeling, 'This is not what I want, though I thought it was.' Only he did not know what he really wanted. To go one step further along this line of reasoning, it may be said that he came to realize that those successes which he had to fight for brought no real satisfaction to his hungry soul, and he longed to be given something without fighting for it. The entry for April 22, 1883, in his diary seems to prove the hypothesis: 'Repented my past sins deeply, and felt my total inability to save myself by my own efforts' (p. 91).

Uchimura spent the next two years in Tokyo trying to find something that could satisfy him. He participated in the Pentecostal services which were quite popular in Tokyo at the time. He also frequently attended parties given by churches. Outwardly his depression might have disappeared for awhile, and it was then that he fell in love with Take Asada, his first wife. In the book he does not mention this very important episode in his life, but the details surrounding the marriage that lasted only for several months and ended in divorce have become clear, thanks to the research done by his biographers. Take was a 'modern' girl, Christian and schooled in the Western style. This was what attracted her to him, but it certainly did not appeal to his old parents, particularly his mother. At one point he gave up the idea of marrying her, but later, encouraged by his friends and with the final though perhaps grudging approval of his parents, he decided to marry her. But once married he found out to his great dismay that he and his bride were not really compatible. Most probably Take irritated him with her too carefree behavior. After some squabble she left him, although he pleaded with her not to. Later when she changed her mind and asked to return, he refused, despite the fact that she was pregnant, and protested that she had been spiritually, if not physically, unfaithful. This sounds self-righteous, but he was serious about it to the end.

The question is why he did not mention this incident in the book. Was it too painful to relate? Undoubtedly. Also, in the light of the depression which he seems to have suffered, his unfortunate marriage and divorce acquires a new meaning. For it seems quite certain that he married out of depression only to sink into it again with the break-up of his marriage. Thus his final rejection of Take, which otherwise might look too cruel, makes sense. Whatever guilt he might have incurred during and after the marriage, it was not, so far as he was concerned, against Take as a person. He must have blamed himself alone for having been too intent on making himself happy by marriage. The unhappy marriage only deepened the sense of disillusionment and guilt which he had been nursing inside for some time. It was in itself a fleeting episode, however painful and tragic. One month after the separation he resigned from a new governmental position he had taken. He then set his mind on going to America. The same impulse which had driven him from Sapporo to Tokyo was with greater force pushing him into an unknown world.

There is one more final note about his failure to mention his first marriage in the book. Its unhappy memory must have naturally weighed heavily on his mind while he was writing the chapter that dealt with this period in his life. Even if he did not specifically mention it, he could not have entirely avoided alluding to it. For instance, when he reflects critically on the prevailing atmosphere in Christian churches during that period – that 'God's kingdom was imagined to be one of perfect repose and constant free exchange of good wishes, where tea-parties and love-makings could be indulged in with the sanction of the religion of free communions and free love' (p. 96), he was undoubtedly thinking of what he had undergone. More important than this is the fact that he put the quotation from Hosea at the head of the chapter. Hosea is known to have had an unhappy married life because of his wife's infidelity, and from this bitter experience he understood the love of God beckoning stray Israel to return to Him. It is most likely that Kanzō chose Hosea because of their common unhappy experience. Most interestingly, however, in the passage that follows the quotation he puts himself in the place of stray Israel, saying, 'So my Lord and Husband must have said to Himself when He drove me from my peaceful home-church' (p. 90). Does this mean that in addition to identifying with Hosea he put himself in the unfaithful wife's place as well? In other words, somewhere deep in his mind he knew, however vaguely, that he was like his wife after all. Or would it be possible to see here an unconscious admission of his original identification with his mother, that he felt an identity as a woman in some strange way? It must be said then that perhaps he revealed himself much more here than had he simply recorded his unhappy marriage.

What roughly corresponds in the life of Luther to this stage in the life of Uchimura is the period stretching from Luther's entry into the University of Erfurt at seventeen to his ordination as a priest at twenty-three. His entry into the monastery comes in between at twenty-one. Referring to his father's curse at the time of his first mass, he later wrote to his father publicly, 'You again hit me so cleverly and fittingly that in my whole life I have hardly heard a word that resounded in me more forcefully and stuck in me more firmly!' (p. 145). What happened then, to quote from Erikson, was as follows: 'Incredible as it seems, at this late date Martin was thrown back into the infantile struggle, not only over his obedience toward, but also over his identification with, his father. This regression and this personalization of his conflict cost him that belief in the monastic way and in his superiors which during the first year had been of such "godly" support' (p. 145).

In other words, he had to combat renewed doubt in his vocation. Thus his scrupulosity, which had found its haven in the monastic life, broke loose, leading to extreme religious preoccupation and erratic behavior which became increasingly noticeable to those around him. His contemporaries reported 'the fit in the choir' among others, in which he suddenly fell to the ground in the choir, 'raved' like one possessed, and roared with the voice of a bull, 'Ich bin's nit! Ich bin's nit!' ('It isn't me!').[14]

This incident took place when the passage from the Bible describing 'Christ's cure of a man possessed by a dumb spirit' was read. Erikson believes that it refers to a story beginning from Mark 9:17, about a certain father who brings to Christ his son possessed by a dumb spirit and given to convulsions. Erikson also intimates that in the very act of denial – 'It isn't me' – Martin revealed his secret identification with the possessed son. Since the fatal reunion with his father, it must have dawned on him that he might be the possessed son after all, an obsession which he desperately fought with all his might.

EXPERIENCES IN AMERICA

Uchimura went to America in November 1884. He states the reason for taking this trip: 'To be a man first and then a patriot, was my aim in going abroad' (p. 102). It is as if he were not yet a man and could not be a patriot in his own country! This clearly supports what has been suggested here, that his unhappy marriage brought home to him anew his basic inadequacy. He found himself in the midst of an identity crisis, not only sexually but socially, for he was completely at a loss about what to make of his future. Hence, his use of the word patriot, for he was yet to find a lifework which could both satisfy him and earn him recognition by his country. But why did he choose to go to America for these purposes, considering financial and other difficulties in making such a trip? About this he says, 'Failing to find the desired satisfaction in my own land, I thought of extending my search to a land differently constituted from my own – even to Christendom, where Christianity having had undisputed power and influence for hundreds of years, must, I imagined, be found Peace and Joy in a measure inconceivable to us of heathen extraction, and easily procurable by any sincere seeker after the Truth' (p. 101).

He clearly felt that his personal difficulties were intricately and mysteriously tied up with his adoption of the Christian belief. He wanted to see with his own eyes what a Christian country was like and also how he would react to such an environment. No sooner had he arrived in America, however, than his hope of finding a superior society was shattered. Free use of profanity, roaming pickpockets, feigned kindness to exploit the unwary, particularly rampant racial prejudice – all these things struck him deeply. He cried, 'O heaven, I am undone! I was deceived! I gave up what was really Peace for that which is no Peace!' (p. 118). He almost regretted having become a Christian. Yet he knew somehow that he had crossed the point of no return. Only, he told himself, he would 'never defend Christianity upon its being the religion of Europe and America' (p. 119).

Soon after his arrival he found employment as an attendant in an insane asylum run by Dr. I. N. Kerlin of Pennsylvania, to whom he was introduced through the wife of M. C. Harris, the missionary who had baptized him. About this employment, Uchimura recalls: 'I took this step, not because I thought the world needed my service in that line, much less did I seek it as an occupation (poor though I was), but because I thought it to be the only refuge from "the wrath to come", there to put my flesh in subjection, and to so discipline myself as to reach the state of inward purity, and thus inherit the kingdom of heaven' (p. 125).

Here looms again the subject of guilt which was tormenting his soul with even stronger force. And I should say it was a well-chosen occupation for a guilt-ridden man. Kerlin on his part, kind and understanding man that he was, sensed the plight of this strange young foreigner and lavished affection on him, at the same time instructing him in the value of medical and philanthropic work. Uchimura felt deep respect and affection for the man and testifies that 'he it was who rescued me from degenerating into that morbid religiosity. . . . Indeed it was he who humanized me' (p. 128). For all his good influence, however, Uchimura could not stay with Kerlin for long. Uchimura knew that he was not cut out for the kind of work he was engaging in, for he was, in his own words, too 'egoistic'. In the meantime 'doubts' within him were becoming 'impossible to be borne for any length of time' (p. 142). At last, after eight months' service, he left for New England.

The reason for his choosing New England as his next destination was obvious: 'I was to see New England by all means, for my Christianity came originally from New England, and she was responsible for all the internal struggles caused thereby' (p. 144). By this he meant that William S. Clark, who originally evangelized Sapporo Agricultural College, came from New England. He reasoned that if there were any place in the world where he could be freed from his internal turmoil, it would be there. It was fortunate for him that J. H. Seeley, president of Amherst College, to whom he was introduced by a friend, gave him an unexpected fatherly welcome and even agreed to accept him as a special student in the junior class. For the first time he felt at ease under the wing of Seeley's protection, however lacking he might have been in material comforts and however lonely without any congenial friends. He states, 'I confess Satan's power over me began to slacken ever since I came in contact with that man' (p. 148).

Through Seeley he gradually came to experience the peace of mind he so much longed for. One day, on March 8, 1886, six months after coming to Amherst, he noted in the diary, 'Very important day in my life. Never was the atoning power of Christ more clearly revealed to me than it is today. In the crucifixion of the Son of God lies the solution of all the difficulties that have buffeted my mind thus far' (p. 153). Later he reported this experience as 'the conciliation of moral schism' (p. 160). The entry for September 13 of the same year is also very moving in that he records a private eucharist he celebrated alone in a dormitory room with juice he pressed out of a cluster of wild grapes and a piece of biscuit. For all his youthful devotion, Christianity had still been something imposed on and not completely assimilated into his soul. But now it was his own. It finally became the substance of himself; he had experienced the wholeness of the faith of Christ.

After completing two years of study at Amherst he entered a theological seminary in Connecticut. From this one might conclude that he had made up his mind to become a Christian minister. But in actuality his decision was a complex one, ridden with doubts and reservations. To become a Christian minister in his day meant to enter the service of a certain denomination whose headquarters existed outside Japan. This his pride could never permit him to undertake. It was completely against the spirit in which he had helped to build Sapporo Independent Church. Also being exposed in America to many denominations all soliciting his allegiance, he was all the more skeptical about belonging to any. He decided that if he must become a Christian minister, he should become an independent one: 'I made up my mind to study Theology, but upon one important condition; and that was that I should never be licensed' (p. 173). With such an unusual decision, how could he have felt at home among seminarians? On the one hand, their worldly ambition to obtain a good position after graduation appalled him. On the other, the academicism in teaching repelled him. And behind all these untoward reactions there lay his mounting nostalgia for Japan. He came to see her good points, which had escaped him before. He even felt that in certain areas Japan might fare more favorably than America. He must have been in agony then as to whether or not he was proceeding on the right path: 'Severe mental strains of the past three years unsettled my nerves, and chronic insomnia of a most fearful kind took hold of me. Rest, bromides, prayers proved ineffectual, and the only way now open for me was one leading toward my homeland' (p. 177). He quit the seminary only a few months after admission and departed for Japan. He arrived there in May 1888. And here the book that traces his spiritual journey up to this point comes to its end.[15]

SUMMING UP

Uchimura left Japan in a state of depression like a fugitive and returned there presumably with a troubled mind which was just as bad, if not worse. In the meantime he experienced a new integration in the faith of Christ and acquired a number of lifelong friends. Among them Seeley stands out as the most important, as he became literally Uchimura's spiritual father. This must have meant a great deal to him, because, as noted earlier, he could not look up to his own father for guidance and protection. He had been without a father spiritually and now was given one. However, except for this experience and other similar ones, his days in America were far from pleasant. I have noted his quick disillusionment with America; it had not been like what his missionary friends in Japan had led him to believe. Then in the final stage of his stay he again had to experience a keen sense of disappointment in his hopes for education in a theological seminary. It was this that made him quit the seminary much too soon and return to Japan earlier than he expected. When he returned, did he feel like a man and a patriot, as he had wished to at the time of going abroad? A man, possibly yes, if his deepened faith made him feel like one. But I rather doubt it. And a patriot he was definitely not, as he was still in the dark as to what would become of him. One might almost say that Uchimura gained his wholeness of faith at the expense of becoming a man and a patriot. Was faith alone then sufficient to him? I doubt this too. I can only imagine how sad and uncertain he must have felt on his return, though he might not have admitted this to others.

I would like to call attention to the curious fact that Uchimura went through one disillusionment after another within a span of five years or so, beginning with the one that originally drove him from Sapporo to Tokyo. And Uchimura was to undergo many more disillusionments in later life. To exaggerate, it is as though he were born to experience disillusionment. Of course everyone will experience disillusionment of one sort or another, some more, others less frequently in life. But in Kanzō's life this stands out as the most prominent feature; it runs through his life as a common thread. And, most interestingly, whether or not he intended it, his book also begins with the theme of disillusionment: 'I was born, according to the Gregorian calendar, on the 28th of March, 1861. My family belonged to the warrior class; so I was born to fight – *vivere est militare* – from the very cradle. My paternal grandfather was every inch a soldier. He was never so happy as when he appeared in his ponderous armour, decked with a bamboo-bow and pheasant-feathered arrows and a 50-pound fire-lock. He lamented that the land was in peace, and died with regret that he never was able to put his trade in practice' (p. 17). (After this comes the description of his father, which I quoted before.)

With this theme of disillusionment as a key concept, I shall make one bold reconstruction of his life. Uchimura as a small child deeply imbibed the feelings of disillusionment and doom that prevailed within his family due to the historical change which drastically altered their fate. His early religiosity, with many superstitious beliefs, can be interpreted as an attempt not to be caught by a fate that threatened to engulf him. Subsequent conversion to Christianity, however, cleared this feeling of impending disaster for him. Thus he could indulge in a feeling of pastoral peace for a while and become absorbed in various activities. But breaking through these defensive activities, the feeling of being doomed once again set in. From that time on he had to fight one disillusionment after another, as if he had to prove that he could survive them all. We shall see how this theory applies to his later life as well.[16]

Now what is a key concept for the life of Luther? It is the theme of justification, as Erikson amply demonstrates from various sources. First, he had to justify his religious vocation in the face of his father's strong opposition to it. Failing this, he would amount to nothing. Unlike Uchimura, he had to fight despair rather than disillusionment, hence his extreme religious and moral scrupulosity. It looks, then, almost like only one more step from such a scrupulosity to his final doctrine of justification only by faith in Christ. True, he found an understanding father figure in Dr. Staupitz, just as Uchimura had in President Seeley. But the contrast in subsequent course between the two is great. Luther held fast until he became a clerical professor of moral philosophy, whereas Uchimura did not even finish theological seminary. Luther was sent to Rome on a business trip as an official representative of his Order, and his ties with the Roman Church were not affected by it. This contrasts sharply with Uchimura's trip to America, where he went with so much hope only to return with a broken heart.

LATER LIFE

In September 1888, soon after Uchimura returned to Japan, he obtained the position of temporary headmaster at a school in Niigata run by foreign missionaries. He resigned it four months later after quarrelling over school policy with the missionaries. This was his first disillusioning experience after his return, and more followed in rapid succession. In September 1890 he became a lecturer at the First Higher School in Tokyo. Four months later he was unexpectedly the center of a scandal: he reportedly hesitated to bow his head in front of the Imperial Rescript on Education, which had the emperor's signature. The rising sentiment of nationalism at once made a traitor out of him, and he had to hand in his resignation under ignominious circumstances. Following this he became gravely ill with pneumonia, and just as he was recovering, his second wife became ill and died.

In a forlorn state of mind he turned to writing, the only means left to him to express himself and possibly earn a living, as he could count on no gainful employment because of the recent scandal. He produced as many as seven books within a few years, one of which was How *I Became a Christian*. It was his way of coming to grips with the terrible misfortune that befell him and also of seeking to define Japan's mission in the world. He was making his name as a Christian author, and he was quite happy with his third marriage. When war broke out between Japan and China in 1894, he championed Japan's cause in a special essay and was rehabilitated from past ignominy at last. He was now proudly a man and a patriot.

It did not take much time, however, before he became disillusioned with Japan, for she acted entirely differently in her war efforts from what he pictured her as doing in his essay. He then decided to start a movement of social reform, joining with like-minded people. He worked for a while as a columnist for *Yorozuchōhō*, an influential newspaper, and founded with his friends the *Tokyo Independent* journal in 1898. This came to an end after two years, when a serious quarrel broke out between him and the other staff, including his brother Tatsusaburō. From this time on he and Tatsusaburō never saw each other. It is also known that his mother and other brothers and sister all took the side of Tatsusaburō against him. I might mention in this connection that his mother became psychotic a few years later and died in an asylum, a fact which aggravated even more the feud between him and his brothers.

In 1900 he founded singlehandedly a monthly journal *Seisho no Kenkyū* (Biblical Studies), which became his lifework and lasted for thirty years until his death. Its publication was soon followed by the opening of a Sunday Bible class, which also lasted until he died. He was now ipso facto an independent Christian minister, though he had no ordination nor church. It was then he coined a new word *Mukyōkai* (Non-church). Interestingly, he declared that it was not meant as a war cry against established churches, but as an invitation to those who did not or could not belong to them for one reason or another. He could have said that Mukyōkai was for those who were disillusioned with or alienated from established churches. At any rate, he never objected to the church institution as such, and besides accepting invitations to speak at many churches he himself occasionally performed baptism and celebrated the eucharist. Thus, the sentiment embodied in his justification for Mukyōkai exactly echoes the defense he once made for the Sapporo Independent Church. While devoting most of his time to missionary work, he still worked as a social critic. But after making the now famous antiwar statement at the time of Russo-Japanese War in 1903, he completely retreated from the public arena and began the life of a full-time Christian minister. By this time he had lost his former passion for social reform. He even began to criticize socialism, the creed of his one-time associates.

The rest of his life was immensely successful and fruitful. His monthly journal of Biblical Studies promised to be successful from the beginning, with its first issue of three thousand copies being sold at once. His influence was nationwide, and the number of his followers increased yearly. Many of them later became national leaders in their respective fields, and some became independent teachers of Christianity like the master. In spite of this great success, disillusionment did not escape him. He had to endure many more bitter experiences, among which I shall mention two as most noteworthy. One was the death of his nineteen-year-old daughter in 1912. When her condition became very grave, it is reported that he prayed to God earnestly to give her a miraculous cure, being firmly convinced that God would listen to his prayer. One can well imagine how deeply disappointed he must have been when he knew that his prayer was not answered. It looks almost as if he were courting disillusionment so that he could overcome it once and for all. After his daughter's death, his faith became very much heaven-bound or eschatological and this, along with his observations on a world that was soon precipitated into The First World War, led to his later movement of the Second Coming of Christ.

The other, also important, source of his disillusionment lay in his relationships with his followers. Some of them whom he loved became apostates later. But it was more painful for him when some of his most trusted assistants disagreed with him on the fundamentals of Christian faith. The most serious conflict occurred toward the end of his life with regard to what Tsukamoto Toraji, his chief assistant who was regarded by all of his followers as his successor, stated as the essence of Christianity. In brief, Tsukamoto attempted to make a logical construct out of Uchimura's life-long teaching that established churches are not only not essential to Christian faith, but harmful. Uchimura vehemently opposed this, saying that his Mukyōkai (Non-church) was not to become an issue in discussing the Christian faith. What he feared most of all was to be looked on as the founder of Tsukamoto's Churchless Christianity, which he instinctively knew would degenerate into another sect, for what he wanted most of all from the beginning was to be independent of any denomination or sect. He could not bear the thought of becoming the founder of a new sect. Soon after virtually excommunicating Tsukamoto, he died a lonely death (on March 28, 1930), leaving word that he wanted to be remembered as having died like a small child clinging to the cross.[17]

Let us now take a look at Luther's life for comparison. The story of how Luther ignited a revolution throughout Europe when he nailed the ninety-five theses on the door of the Castle Church in Wittenberg in 1517 is so well known that it does not have to be retold. Luther did not dream of a complete break with the Roman Church at the beginning. He only wanted to cleanse the Church of its abuses. But he gradually became involved with the political and social upheaval he helped to stir up, and found himself at a point of no return in his open revolt against the Roman Church, so that he had to establish his own separate church. In all this he vehemently justified his actions, but soon the reaction to it came in the form/shape of a severe depression. Then he was unable to believe his own justification of himself, even by faith, as he proclaimed. It is known that he suffered from such depression periodically until he died at sixty-three in 1546. This quick glance at his later life may be sufficient to distinguish it from Uchimura's. After having lived in a cloistered monastery for over ten years, Luther was a most important public figure throughout most of his adult life whereas Uchimura engaged as a journalist in a social movement or national politics only for a short while, and soon after retreated from all this, devoting himself totally to his religious mission. Luther established his own church, whereas Uchimura did not even appoint his successor, refusing to see the birth of a sect in his time.

CONCLUSION

Among Christian Thinkers[18]

Christianity is a religion which claims universalism. As St. Paul said, 'There is one Lord, one faith, one baptism, and one God who is Father of all, over all, through all, and within all' (Ephesians 4:5-6). However, from the beginning of Christianity there was a strong tendency to diversification or even dissension due to personal or regional factors, as can be seen from a reading of the New Testament books. Still, the canonization of the New Testament books in the early period of Christianity indicates an attempt to integrate such diverse views, that is, a manifestation of universalism. This dialectical movement of two opposing tendencies, unification and diversification, runs through the entire history of Christianity to this day.

What attracted Uchimura Kanzō to Christianity was its professed universalism. But it was not long before he was exposed to its diverse denominations. His American experience further taught him a lesson that what goes in the name of Christianity is not necessarily Christian. Then in his subsequent struggle to grasp the essence of Christianity he was gradually led to discover the worth of his Japanese heritage: '. . . looking at a distance from the land of my exile, my country ceased to be a "good-for-nothing". It began to appear superbly beautiful – not the grotesque beauty of my heathen days, but the harmonic beauty of true proportions, occupying a definite space in the universe with its own historic individualities' (p. 122). It is not that he placed the Japanese heritage above Christianity. He felt, however, that he had a special advantage as a Japanese in appreciating Christianity, and Japan should have a mission of her own in the scheme of God.

Uchimura wrote the following words on the back of the cover of his Bible while he was studying at Amherst College: 'To be inscribed upon my Tomb. I for Japan; Japan for the World; The World for Christ; And All for God.' This clearly shows that he felt responsible for the conversion of the nation just as he once felt for the conversion of his family. Thus it became his lifework to present pure Christianity, or one might say orthodox Christianity, to the Japanese people. As he did so, his Christian beliefs and thinking inevitably took a certain shape which distinguishes him from Christian thinkers in the West. I shall try here to compare his position with that of some of the most prominent figures in the history of Christianity.

First, Uchimura shared with St. Paul a strong conviction of being chosen as the minister of the word of God. They were probably similar in temperament, both being passionate fighters. They were also deeply troubled by quarrels among Christians. St. Paul in his first letter to Corinthians admonishes them over fighting among themselves, presumably about who was baptized by whom, and states 'Christ did not send me to baptize, but to preach the Good News.' These words must have rung true for Uchimura. However, there was an important difference between the two in their dealing with division among Christians. St. Paul firmly believed in the unity of the Church, whereas Uchimura tried to dispense with churches and invented the notion of Mukyōkai (Non-church). One might say that Uchimura's notion of church was sociological rather than theological.

Second, Uchimura shared with Augustine a pagan background, and both left the record of their conversion for the benefit of posterity. But the ways in which they were converted were quite different. In the case of Augustine, his mother had been a Christian and his father a pagan. He tried to escape the influence of his mother, who wanted to make a Christian out of him, and, fleeing her and Christianity, finally reached a point where he could no longer resist becoming a Christian. It was a long spiritual journey with many detours. In the case of Uchimura, Christianity with its accompanying Western culture was forced on him as something far superior to what he had before. So his real struggle began after he was converted. It was the struggle to make Christianity his own. He finally made it, but then he was not quite sure of his standing. Surely he prided himself on his independence, but it cost him life-long suffering, as he was fraught with conflicts over deeply buried dependency wishes. None of his father figures – let alone his own father, or even Seeley who helped him greatly – represented a true authority with which he could identify. For one thing, this was because the type of Puritan Christianity he espoused was no longer a dominant force in American society. Augustine, while not able to identify with his pagan father, could identify himself with the authority of the growing Catholic Church and thereby be saved from being dominated by his mother and at the same time reconciled with her. Thus he became one of the most important spiritual fathers in the history of Christianity. Uchimura was never happy with the fatherly role, refusing to be a father even to his closest disciples.

Third, Uchimura shares with Luther morbidly intense guilt feelings. But the circumstances which led to such an overwrought conscience were different between the two. In the case of Luther the guilt was originally implanted by his much too severe parents. His choice of monastic life was a compromise, on the one hand, of the guilt he imbibed from theirs and, on the other, a rebellion against his father, who had decided on a secular career for him. But as he could not succeed in appeasing his father, his guilt became intensified until he found for himself justification by faith in Christ. It was by historical accident that he found himself in open revolt against the papacy – a most opportune outlet for his long smouldering fury. In leaving the monastery behind, he became a historical figure who ushered in a new era, finally meeting his father's original expectations of him. Still he would not give credit to his father! One may say that Luther became his own father by eliminating all father figures available on earth. In theological terms, he identified both with Christ and His Father. This Uchimura would never do, as he remained at heart a small lonely child until the end of his life.

Fourth, Uchimura and Pascal were both scientists turned religious thinkers, but they differed considerably in relating their scientific Weltanschauung to Christian beliefs. Perhaps this was because Uchimura was a scientist only by training, whereas Pascal was a great scientist who shaped modern science. Still, the difference in their conceptions of science *vis-à-vis* religion is remarkable. For Pascal, science was an autonomous domain of human knowledge which was totally independent of religion. One might say that in this respect he was even more Cartesian than Descartes himself. His expression, 'the eternal silence of these infinite spaces terrifies me' foresees the terror of modern man left alone with nothing but science. This sentiment was completely missing in Uchimura. His Christian belief was inseparable from a belief in God as the Creator of all. God was not hidden for him as for Pascal; no dichotomy of science and religion existed. Thus, Uchimura welcomed natural science wholeheartedly, for it helped him to appreciate God all the more as the Creator. Should one say that Uchimura was naive? Perhaps he was, but he certainly was more biblical in this respect. He could perceive the fruits of reason as a blessing (a notion forgotten in the West) precisely because he was naive as a good Japanese should be.

Fifth, Uchimura shared with Kierkegaard a determined refusal to be officially ordained as a minister because of the unique mission each felt destined to fulfill. Uchimura's mission was to bring pure Christianity to Japan, whereas Kierkegaard's was to make the post-Christian age again ready for Christianity. Both suffered periods of depression, which was related to their original experience of Christianity. Uchimura felt that Christianity created new problems for him which it did not solve. For Kierkegaard the crisis which he called the great earthquake came with his growing realization that his religious father, who used to share imaginary trips with him as a child, was in reality a spiritually dead man obsessed with memories of past sins and the idea of impending disaster as a divine punishment. After having been completely immersed in his father's melancholy, he tried to extricate himself from it by vigorously engaging in intellectual life and eventually discovering for himself and others true Christianity. In this process he saw the falsity and emptiness of what ordinarily passed for Christianity, just as he had seen his father's religiosity as impotent. He was perhaps a more unhappy and lonelier man than Uchimura, for he remained single and never formed a group of followers. Uchimura was a self-appointed minister, but Kierkegaard could not permit himself to be one, committing his thoughts only to writing. When he finally plunged into action, he charged like a madman, vehemently attacking official Christianity in public, dying a few months later of exhaustion. It seems then that for all his penetrating insights into Christianity, psychology, and the present age, he was never entirely freed from his father's melancholy.

Sixth, Uchimura can be likened to Bonhoeffer, for his notion of Mukyōkai is very close to what Bonhoeffer spelled out as religionless Christianity. Uchimura is reported to have often said, 'Christianity is not a religion',[19] and in that case his idea and Bonhoeffer's almost become identical. One difference between the two is that for Uchimura the notion of Mukyōkai was a kind of springboard without which he could not have started his mission. It was his point of departure. For Bonhoeffer the notion of religionless Christianity was his terminal point. In his student days he once visited Rome and was deeply impressed by the Catholic Church. Because of this experience, when he became a full-fledged minister he devoted most of his talent and energy to the task of building up the Confessing Church to which he belonged. This became an urgent matter when the Nazi persecution of churches began. After fighting a losing battle in his attempt to consolidate the Confessing Church against the Nazis, he committed himself to the anti-Nazi movement, but soon was arrested and finally hanged. It was during prison life that he developed a notion of religionless Christianity. He mused on what Christians could do in this godless, religionless world, and came to the conclusion that they could not and should not rely on whatever was left of man's need for religion, and they themselves should be able to get by without such a need, only participating in the sufferings of God at the hands of a godless world. Clearly Bonhoeffer was disillusioned with existing churches, just as Uchimura was. It is interesting to note in this regard that Bonhoeffer's family and its close circle were not particularly religious, though very cultured, loving, and definitely anti-Nazi. His father Karl was a famous professor of psychiatry at the University of Berlin. One could say then that with the idea of religionless Christianity, Bonhoeffer's original identification with his family stood out clearly, as his hope for and identification with the Confessing Church became very faint in his last days.[20]

The Japanese Heritage in Uchimura

As the preceding comparison indicates, one can draw parallels between Uchimura and Christian thinkers in the West. Yet there is something about his life and work that can be attributed only to his Japanese heritage. To stress this point, I shall take up his keen sense of disillusionment, his neglect of things institutional, and the kind of sect he helped to create.

First, there is no doubt that he was particularly sensitive to disillusionment. It was, in my opinion, due to his identification with his disillusioned father and at the same time to what he missed in his early relationship with his mother. It was his mother, not his father, who became a formidable parent with whom he had to deal. Such a family constellation is not rare in Japan; in fact I would say that his was not so uncommon a case. What was remarkable was that he created a historical role for himself out of the sense of disillusionment. Mukyōkai was meant for those disillusioned with established churches, and it appealed strongly to those who were disillusioned for other reasons as well. This explains why Uchimura had a special attraction for Japanese intellectuals, because they were the ones most dissatisfied with Japanese society. Thus he became a kind of father-figure for them, even though in his personal relations he was not really happy with the father role.[21]

Second, Uchimura was immensely successful as a lay preacher, and his neglect of institutions appealed to many sensitive Japanese, who tended to perceive institutions as something external to themselves, hence lifeless. True, Uchimura occasionally performed the rite of baptism or eucharist when he found it appropriate to do so, in spite of his frequently voiced opinion that the sacraments were not essential for faith. This looks like a contradiction, but he never bothered to explain it. And the fact that he never bothered is superb proof that he regarded institutions or sacraments only from a viewpoint of expediency.

Third, as described here, Uchimura rightly refused to have his idea of Mukyōkai institutionalized. Yet he could not prevent his followers from forming a sect, which consisted of a number of separate groups, each tightly knit around a single teacher. This was a style he himself created. And he created it, I should say, because he was a passionate advocate of friendship and discipleship. Also, as has been hinted here, there is reason to believe that his Mukyōkai mission was a late product of what originally prompted him to establish a church in his Sapporo days. Therefore it would not be too far-fetched to say that the Mukyōkai sect was an institutionalization of friendship and discipleship, two virtues highly appreciated in Japanese society. It is because of this that only in this sect, among the many Christian churches, does male attendance usually outnumber female. But then why did Uchimura not pride himself on the creation of such a sect? Why did he not acknowledge it?

I have noted here that Uchimura yielded to group pressure in accepting a new faith and as a consequence was subjected to severe internal turmoil.

This incidentally represents a typical pattern which has been repeated numerous times in Japan whenever a new ideology is introduced. It usually starts with a small coterie of new adherents which accumulates momentum by virtue of group attraction until it becomes a sizable clique. To step out of one's group after initial identification with it is extremely difficult for Japanese, and many are wrecked in that process, as recent student movements attest. Perhaps Uchimura knew all this instinctively. That is why he came to value his independence more than anything else, and also why he never tried to hold back those who wanted to leave him. He demanded independence of his followers. Is this possibly what was in back of his mind when he refused to see the birth of a new sect in his name? He would not yield to or condone group pressure in his last days as he had earlier. In other words, Uchimura as a person was far above the Mukyōkai sect he helped to create. Therein lies his true greatness.

NOTES

1.　Uchimura Kanzō, *How I Became a Christian. Complete Works of Uchimura Kanzō*, vol. 1 (Tokyo: Kyōbunkan, 1971). Page references to this volume are noted directly in the text.
2.　Erik H. Erikson, *Young Man Luther* (New York: Norton, 1958).
3.　*Amae* is the noun form derived from *amaeru*, a unique Japanese verb which signifies a desire for love or behavior indicating such a desire. See Doi Takeo's *The Anatomy of Dependence* (Tokyo: Kodansha International, 1973).
4.　Uchimura Miyoko, who was a devoted disciple of Uchimura Kanzō and later married his son, Yūshi, gives a vivid picture of his personality in her memoir on Kanzō (*Kanzō yakyū seishinigaku*, Tokyo: Nihon Keizai Shimbun Sha, 1973). Her story supports the inference about Kanzō not being favored by his mother. She told me in private conversation that his mother favored his brother Tatsusaburō, a fact which contributed to a future quarrel between the two brothers, as will be discussed later. She also remembers Kanzō's statement when his mother died: 'How sad that I must do a funeral for a mother who never loved me.' This explains Kanzō's life-long search for the loving mother figure. Again according to Uchimura Miyoko, Kanzō depended very much on his wife, and toward the end of his life particularly enjoyed the company of a few women followers.
5.　Erikson, *Young Man Luther*, p. 91.
6.　*Ibid.*, pp. 64 and 67-68.
7.　*Ibid.*, pp. 65 and 67.
8.　About the Japanese custom of solving ambivalence by playing *omote* and *ura* alternately, see Doi Takeo's article, '*Omote* and *Ura*: Concepts Derived from the Japanese Two-Fold Structure of Consciousness', *Journal of Nervous and Mental Disease*, vol. 154, no. 4 (1973), pp. 258-261. To explain it in brief, *omote* stands for the surface that can be shown to others, and *ura* for what has to be kept in back of one's mind or can be confided only to those very close to oneself. Japanese are taught from early years to distinguish between the two, which actually make up the backbone of Japanese morality. Uchimura's failure to acquiesce in the seeming discrepancy between the two modes of conduct again bespeaks his lack of maternal love, because it is the mother who usually habituates children to such dealings.
9.　Erikson, *Young Man Luther*, p. 92.
10.　*Ibid.*, p. 144.
11.　*Ibid.*, p. 145.
12.　*Ibid.*, p. 146.

13. 'Some Character Types Met with in Psychoanalytic Work' (1916), *Complete Psychological Works of Sigmund Freud*, vol. 14 (London: Hogarth, 1957), pp. 316-331.
14. Erikson, *Young Man Luther*, p. 23.
15. It is known that Kanzō even after he returned to Japan and until his death continued to suffer from insomnia, and that he also had attacks of anxiety from time to time. This indicates that, along with his history of early religious scrupulosity and subsequent depression, he was never completely freed from conflicts over *amae*, not withstanding his firm Christian beliefs. Or rather it may be said that his Christian beliefs even intensified his conflicts, though they certainly helped him overcome his early polytheistic attachments. It seems to be in the nature of religion to make psychic conflicts more accessible or active so that they must be dealt with (successfully or unsuccessfully).
16. It is interesting to note in this regard that the first book he wrote was titled *Kirisuto shinto no nagusame* (The Christian's Consolations).
17. Yamamoto Taijirō, *Uchimura Kanzō-Shinkō, Shōgai, Yūjō* (Tokyo: Tōkai Daigaku Shuppankai, 1966), p. 290.
18. In preparing this section I was helped by the following books, among others: Augustine's *Confessions*; Erikson's *Young Man Luther*; Pascal's *Pensées*; Walter Lowrie's *A Short Life of Kierkegaard* (New York: Doubleday Anchor, 1961); Mary Bosanquet's *Life and Death of Dietrich Bonhoeffer* (New York: Harper Colophon, 1973).
19. Yamamoto, *Uchimura Kanzō*, pp. 169, 228.
20. Another coincidence between Bonhoeffer and Uchimura is that Bonhoeffer's father Karl and Uchimura's son Yūshi were both psychiatrists. Yūshi is now professor emeritus at the University of Tokyo.
21. It seems that most of the spiritual leaders in Japan underwent some terribly disillusioning experience to reach a certain enlightenment. This sharply contrasts with the West, where spiritual leaders are usually men of vision. This trend might be attributed to the influence of Buddhism, but I would rather think that it has more to do with the psychology of *amae* which pervades Japanese society. In this regard, see Natsume Sōseki's novel *Kokoro*, in which the chief character called Sensei (meaning master or teacher) is a very impressive person not only to the young man in the story but also to readers. But he is in actuality a terribly disillusioned man bordering on psychosis and eventually commits suicide (compare Doi Takeo's *The Psychological World of Natsume Sōseki*, Harvard University Press, 1976).

It was Uchimura's tragedy that although he became an awe-inspiring and influential teacher he was not happy in the father role, as can be seen from his stressful relationship with his disciples. Furthermore, there is reason to believe that his relationship with his own son was also a strained one. Discretion forbids me to quote his son's remarks on the matter.

First published in Paul B. Pederson, Norman Sartorius, Anthony J. Marsella (Eds), *Mental Health Services – The Cross-Cultural Context*, Sage Publications, 1984

⑯ Psychotherapy – A Cross-cultural Perspective from Japan

This chapter attempts a cross-cultural perspective on psychotherapy. The rationale that calls for such a perspective at the present time is as follows. First, it is now widely acknowledged that all kinds of psychotherapy are deeply rooted in the culture of their origin. This can be said not only of clearly culture-bound psychotherapy, such as Morita therapy in Japan or some folk therapies in developing countries, but also of admittedly culture-free psychotherapy such as psychoanalysis. Second, because of the insight into the cultural origin of various forms of psychotherapy, a new awareness has developed of the necessity for cultural sensitivity within psychotherapy, that is to say, cross-cultural psychotherapy, particularly when the therapist and the patient do not come from the same cultural background. Third, there is, nonetheless, a seemingly opposite trend to this new awareness, since certain originally esoteric forms of psychotherapy may find a clientele among a population that is not related to the culture of their origin. One can immediately call to mind as an example the recent vogue of transcendental meditation in certain parts of the United States. In the same vein, one may interpret the fact that Western-based psychoanalysis finds adherents in non-Western countries such as Japan or India.

This crossing of psychotherapy beyond its original cultural boundary may not be surprising, however, if one considers the facts that today, compared with previous ages, an increasing number of people are crossing from one culture to another and that cultures themselves are undergoing changes due to influences from extraneous cultures. As a matter of fact, it is not infrequent nowadays, especially in the United States, that a person coming from a completely different culture serves as psychiatrist in a host culture, or even becomes a professor of psychiatry, teaching neophytes the trade of psychotherapy. Furthermore, during the past several decades, cultural mixing has occurred at an accelerated pace at the level of culture itself as well as among various populations. This coincides significantly with the mushrooming of new brands of psychotherapy as well as the keen interest shown by various disciplines in the cultural aspects of psychotherapy (Marsella, Tharp, & Cibrowski, 1979; Lebra, 1976; Pedersen,

Draguns, Lonner, & Trimble, 1981). With these factors in mind, it is all the more urgent to have a clear perspective on the relationship between psychotherapy and culture.

Before I proceed to the main points of my discussion, a few words are necessary about the type of approach I will take. I have said that this chapter offers a cross-cultural perspective on psychotherapy. I want to emphasize that it is a perspective, not an overview of all the pertinent literature on the subject. In order to have a perspective, one must ascertain where one stand *vis-à-vis* the particular subject one is investigating and how one came to that view, for these are the very things that decide the kind of perspective one achieves. In other words, any perspective must be personal. So, in presenting my perspective, let me briefly state my background in order to clarify the point from which I shall proceed.

THE POINT OF PERSPECTIVE

I was born in Japan and educated there through medical school, from which I graduated in 1942. I later had the good fortune to study in the United States, first for two years (from 1950 to 1952) and, after a five-year interval, for yet another year. Prior to this, I was already interested in the psychological problems the patients almost invariably presented in my medical practice during the postwar years. At the time, I did not know what to do with them, since I had been taught nothing about them in my medical education. So I avidly read as many articles in American journals as I could obtain that dealt with such problems as I was faced with in my practice. Naturally, I was very happy when the opportunity arose to study in the United States. It was a great learning experience for me in many ways, because it was the first time that I experienced a culture completely different from my own. What was most important for my subsequent career was the full exposure to a psychoanalytic psychiatry that was diametrically different from the prewar German school of psychiatry that I had learned in medical school.

At that time, psychoanalysis was at the peak of its popularity in the United States. Actual exposure to this fact aroused my curiosity as to why psychoanalysis was so popular in the United States, apparently more so than in Europe where it originated, and also made me wonder why it did not fire fervor in Japan, for Freud's ideas had been introduced through the Japanese translation of his main works in the early part of this century. My attention was also called to Morita therapy as a unique Japanese psychotherapy and I was struck by a peculiar difference between this and psychoanalysis, not only in terms of therapeutic procedures or theories behind them, but what these two regarded as suitable cases for their treatment methods. Psychoanalysis began with treatment of hysterical cases, whereas Morita therapy began with hypochondriacal cases. Each specifically regarded as unsuitable for its treatment method that which the other regarded as suitable. At least, those were Freud's and Morita's position, respectively, when they began their work.

These questions have haunted me and still do to a certain extent. It was in grappling with these questions that my own theory of *amae* was developed; I have written a great deal about *amae* both in Japanese and English (Doi, 1962, 1963, 1973a). I shall mention a few points here that directly concern the questions I raised above. First, for Japanese people as a whole, dependency need is readily admitted to one's consciousness as well as subjected to control by the kind of interpersonal relationships one enters, while for Americans it seems to be altogether repressed or denied. On the one hand we find among Japanese the existence of a unique concept of *amae* denoting the satisfaction of such a need and a related vocabulary to describe its manifestations in various situations, including its frustration; among Americans, on the other hand, we find the idealization of individual freedom and independence.

Second, it was perhaps because it catered to the wish to determine one's own destiny that psychoanalysis became popular in the United States, for, according to its doctrines, one controls one's destiny by mastering one's unconscious. Thus psychoanalysis helps promote in the minds of those who engage in it the precious illusion of control over fate, that is, the sense of autonomy. In Japan, on the other hand, it could never have hoped to become popular precisely because in the Japanese ethos one is taught always to take into account fate, which shapes one's destiny. Undoubtedly, this difference in attitudes toward fate is related to the difference in the attitudes toward dependency need. One may say that dependency need by definition all but precludes autonomy, for it is contingent for its satisfaction on so many factors one cannot control – in short, on fate.

Third, Morita therapy succeeded where psychoanalysis failed, presumably because in Morita therapy the problems of dependency are dealt with intuitively. However, it is only in recent years that psychoanalysis came to grips conceptually with these problems. It would appear that the Japanese experience concerning dependency need, in addition to being an expression of Japanese culture, can claim universal validity. In fact, it is my understanding that such a view may release psychoanalysis from its culture-specific underpinnings and strengthen it as a universal theory.

A THEORETICAL MODEL FOR PSYCHOTHERAPY

I think from the beginning my impulse has been to seek a unified theory for psychotherapy, though I have been fully aware of the existing cultural differences. This impulse has been further stimulated by the development during the past few decades of many new psychotherapeutic methods, which I suspect were the result of social and cultural changes in recent years. In short, I have wanted to bring a certain order to the chaos that has overtaken the field of psychotherapy and have sincerely thought that it would also serve the purpose of consolidating the psychiatrist's position in this expanding field. Many have attempted a similar venture, apparently with the same motive (Karasu, 1977; Neil & Ludwig, 1980; Ellenberger, 1982; Havens, 1981); mine appeared in a short paper titled 'Psychotherapy as Hide-and-Seek' (Doi, 1973b), in which I proposed that the children's game of hide-and-seek, and its earlier form, peek-a-boo, consisting of alternate disappearing and reappearing, serves as a theoretical model for all kinds of psychotherapy, ancient and modern, Eastern and Western. It is difficult to say why I hit upon this idea. All I can say is that I must have been led to this proposition from three premises: first, that all forms of psychotherapy are based upon the interpersonal relationship; second, dependency need is instrumental in inducing the interpersonal relationship or object relations at infancy or even in later years, hence it should also underlie the psychotherapeutic relationship; third, the measure of dependency need that operates in the psychotherapeutic relationships can be adequately characterized by hide-and-seek and peek-a-boo.

Hide-and-seek can be played only by those children who have established object relations, whereas peek-a-boo is more appropriate for those who are in the process of developing object relations. In psychotherapy, the patient is urged to engage in either or both of the two following activities: namely, to explore the hidden psyche that is the cause of his or her trouble and to be reassured and comforted by the presence of the therapist on whom the patient comes to depend. It appears that the former process is hide-and-seek and the latter is peek-a-boo. I think this model of hide-and-seek and peek-a-boo for psychotherapy can be further simplified, for there is definitely a developmental continuum from peek-a-boo to hide-and-seek and both are based on the dichotomous pattern of familiar-unfamiliar that emerges in early infancy. This aspect of infant development has been investigated by Bowlby (1971) and others, but I shall not go into details here. It will suffice to point out that all kinds of psychotherapy take after the patterns of familiar-unfamiliar, because, just as the infant is drawn toward the familiar and avoids or is alarmed by what is strange, psychotherapy in any form attempts to make whatever threatens the patient innocuous and acceptable. Let us see in detail how this model fits in with all forms of psychotherapy.

PSYCHOTHERAPIES IN VIEW OF THE ABOVE MODEL

I shall enumerate various kinds of psychotherapy to see if each can be explained by the above model. In psychoanalysis one has to be sufficiently secure to embark on a lonely journey, albeit with the help of the analyst, seeking a pathogenic secret in one's hidden psyche. Thus psychoanalysis is hide-and-seek within one's own person. Exploratory psychotherapy other than orthodox psychoanalysis may be included in this category. Compared to this kind of psychotherapy, supportive psychotherapy is essentially peek-a-boo, inasmuch as one is reassured and comforted by the presence of others, thus being strengthened and confirmed in one's vital ties with others. I think both exploratory and supportive psychotherapy can be nicely summed up by the familiar-unfamiliar pattern as was hinted above. That is, in the former the pathogenic material is pathogenic precisely because it is perceived as foreign to oneself and has to be drawn out in order to make it more to one's liking; in the latter the familiar side of personality is to be reinforced *vis-à-vis* the unfamiliar world.

It is interesting to note here that the conceptual distinction between explorative and supportive psychotherapy, though it may be blurred in actual practice, is peculiar to those Western societies in which the tenets of psychoanalysis are accepted. It goes without saying also that psychoanalysis in its individualistic form could develop only in the Western world. As for supportive psychotherapy, the story is a bit complicated and I shall come back to this later. Now, what I would like to emphasize here is the fact that in all non-Western psychotherapies the explorative aspect and the supportive aspect are always intermingled, that is, not separated as in Western societies. Take shamanism or religious healing, for instance. What troubles the person is divined by the shaman, a process that somewhat resembles explorative psychotherapy in the Western world. But what is noteworthy is that this act takes place usually in the public or within a setting of communal living. Particularly in primitive societies it is a rule that the whole congregation participates in the healing process, thus helping the afflicted one to be restored to his or her proper place in society. This aspect of shamanism undoubtedly corresponds to supportive psychotherapy in the Western world.

Interestingly, this blending of the explorative and the supportive also applies to Morita therapy and Naikan therapy, the methods of treatment developed in modern Japan. I shall not try to belabor this point here, since both therapies are well described in English (Kondo, 1976; Murase, 1976) and the above point is apparent to anyone who has read about those therapies. I would also like to add that the distinction between the explorative and the supportive does not apply either to behavioral or to existential therapy, though the model of psychotherapy I have proposed above applies equally to both: Namely, the learning that is so much emphasized in behavioral therapy is to make what is unfamiliar familiar and the experience that supposedly promotes personal growth in existential therapy is predicated upon the genuine familiarity shared by therapist and patient.

Therefore, the theoretical model I have proposed fits in very well with any form of psychotherapy and gives some order to so confused and fluid a field as psychotherapy. Furthermore, it solves the question of cultural varieties in psychotherapy at one stroke, for culture is what is shared by the members of a community as familiar. Naturally, it differs from culture to culture. But then the question arises as to whether or not psychotherapy is the same as culture learning, that is to say, ordinary education. Certainly, it may not be unreasonable to place psychotherapy within the broader category of education. One may note in this regard that Freud (1963) called psychoanalytic treatment a kind of after-education. But the further question arises as to why psychoanalysis and other schools of psychother- apy developed particularly in nineteenth-century Europe. Why do they still flourish and proliferate in the contemporary world? It is to these questions that I will now turn.

PSYCHOTHERAPY AND CULTURAL CONFLICTS

I shall begin by asking whether there is any special characteristic that distinguishes psychotherapy from ordinary culture learning or accultura- tion. The answer to this question involves the very problems of culture, because, in ordinary culture learning, culture itself is never questioned – it is taken for granted. Psychotherapy is indicated where culture itself has to be questioned, specifically, when the internalization of the conflicting cultural values disturbs one's familiar world, making one part of the self strange to another, thus leading to alienation from the self.

The internalization of the conflicting cultural values is not the same as the concept of instinctual conflict that Freud made so much use of in his theory of neuroses. However, it is possible to interpret the instinctual conflict as a result of cultural conflicts, since the instinctual conflict necessarily involves cultural values. Or, taking the instinctual conflict to be basic to psychopathology, as Freud did, one can see that the existence of conflicts resulting from the clash of different cultural values weakens the hold of the cultural regulations over instinctual drives, thus leading to the instinctual conflict. At any rate, it is logical to assume that the existence of conflicts precedes the development of psychopathology, which is the object of psychotherapy. It follows that the main task of psychotherapy is to identify whatever conflict afflicts the person, then to isolate it in order to prevent it from affecting the whole person and if possible to heal the division within the person. I think that focusing upon the conflict within the afflicted person is most deliberately dealt with in psychoanalysis and its related schools. I should think that the same process takes place inadvertently in other schools of psychotherapy as well, that is, apart from the therapist's intention, even in behavioral and existential therapies.

Now if what distinguishes psychotherapy from ordinary culture learning lies in the preexistence of cultural conflicts, it becomes easier to answer the question of why the important schools of psychotherapy developed in nineteenth-century Europe. As van den Berg (1974) illustrates by many examples in his historical and sociocultural studies, there is no doubt that the development of modern psychotherapies is related to the profound changes in Europe during the past centuries, which culminated in disruption of its traditional unity, thus generating conflicts in various spheres of society. In this regard, one may well understand the notion of anomie formulated by Emile Durkheim. I once addressed the same question with regard to psychoanalysis in one of my papers:

> It is well to remember here, however, that at the time when psychoanalysis

was first invented by Freud the cataclysm of the Western world was already under way. One can recall in this regard names like Nietzsche and Kierkegaard. Is not the development of psychoanalysis also related to this cultural and social crisis? Heinz Hartmann [1958], reflecting on the question of why psychoanalysis emerged at the time it did, stated as follows: 'Apparently at certain points in history the ego can no longer cope with its environment, particularly not with that which it itself has created: the means and goal of life lose their orderly relation, and the ego then attempts to fulfill its organizing function by increasing its insight into the inner world.' In other words, psychoanalysis was an attempt of the ego to re-collect itself *vis-à-vis* the demoralizing world. (Doi, 1964, p. 13)

The above thesis, which relates the development of modern psychotherapies to historical changes, can be equally stated about the cases of Morita therapy and Naikan therapy in Japan. Both came into existence in the present century, presumably because a large number of Japanese people who were undergoing modernization and its accompanying cultural conflicts suffered from neuroses and needed special help. This is evident in Morita therapy, where the patient is repeatedly reassured of the normality and naturalness of his or her socially untoward reactions, and in Naikan therapy, where the patient is urged to recollect his or her so far unacknowledged debts to close relatives. Remember that the features emphasized in these therapies are the things that tend to be overlooked in the inhumanly competitive life of the contemporary world. It is for this reason that these therapies help the patients recover the lost balance of their minds, which initiated their mental sufferings.

Furthermore, there is good reason to believe that the folk therapies in so-called primitive societies (at least some of them) may also be a reaction to the crises caused by the intrusion of Western civilization into their world. Prince (1979) cites two examples: a new type of healing shrine among the rural Ashanti and other groups in response to the disorganizing effects of Westernization (described by M. J. Field) and the healing sessions in Iquitos by culturally mixed populations undergoing rapid culture changes. I suspect that if one examines developing countries more carefully, one may find more examples of this kind. For instance, the cargo cult in Melanesia, which has been reported since the late nineteenth century, may be another such example. This is a cult that expects the resolution of social, political, and economic problems all at once by the arrival of an imaginary cargo full of wealth. Burton-Bradley (1975, p. 16), who studies the culture extensively, states:

Cargo anxiety is the essential feature of many instances of pathological anxiety in Melanesia. It is essentially a status anxiety which arises from imbalance between the forces making for development and those of the status quo. It is the consequence of cultural encounter. It permeates almost all aspects of life, often in covert or subdued form, and it embellishes the symptomatology of many forms of psychiatric disorder. . . . Each patient is a real or potential cargo leader, fortuitously cut short in the course of his career.

Incidentally, the same logic may be applied to the syncretistic aspects of shamanistic religions noted by various scholars. It is likely that they resulted from the efforts to cope with induced cultural changes. Thus the fact of syncretism is the historical residue of cultural changes, though the shamans, in the apt phrase of Hippler (1976, p. 103), simply 'change their tactics with their cultural milieu'. I assume that the same mechanism might have operated behind the famous syncretism in the ancient Mediterranean civilization as well as the similar phenomena manifested in the history of religions in Japan. To pursue this line of argument, however, would be beyond the scope of this chapter.

THE SUPPORTIVE FUNCTION OF PSYCHOTHERAPY IN THE PRESENT AGE

When one surveys the developments in psychotherapy during the past few decades, one cannot help but be struck by an emerging emphasis on its supportive function. I think it was during the 1950s, when psychoanalysis was most prestigious and idealized in the minds of many professionals, that one began hearing about supportive psychotherapy. It was then thought of only as a second best for those cases that were not amenable to the strict psychoanalytic approach. Lately, however, this attitude has considerably changed and supportive psychotherapy has grown steadily in importance, so much so that even in psychoanalysis there is now mention of its supportive function. For this one may refer to the parental component in the analyst's identity, according to Stone (1961), or the holding environment provided by the analyst, according to Winnicott (1965). If one looks beyond the narrow confines of individual psychoanalysis, the emphasis on the supportive function of psychotherapy is too obvious to attract attention. But how else would one explain a new popularity of group psychotherapy or family therapy? The spread of the therapeutic community approach may also bespeak the same trend. More significantly, whenever the therapeutic strategy for each patient is discussed at clinical conferences, one would invariably hear whether the patient's support system is adequate or needs reinforcement. The success of 'crisis intervention' hinges upon whether or not the patient's support system can be mobilized speedily and effectively.

I think this emphasis on the supportive function of psychotherapy can easily be interpreted as a response to a widely felt need in the contemporary world. In the present age, because of wars, revolutions, and unprecedented changes caused by advanced technology, many people feel increasingly insecure, dislocated, and exposed to unknown dangers, as everywhere the familiar world appears to be shrinking ever more rapidly. Terms such as 'pluralism' or 'cultural relativism' are only academic euphemisms; they may soothe the minds of intellectuals, but ordinary people would prefer to flock to whatever promises them protection from the unknown menace they intuitively sense. Hence the development of new therapies in both advanced and developing countries as a kind of shelter from the unfamiliar world. In this connection, it may be interesting to note the new rise in occultism or superstitious beliefs in advanced countries, which is evidence that the recognition of 'fate', which had hitherto been breezily disavowed, is once again assuming a position of importance in the minds of people.

I would like to mention in passing that the character of the present age has been noticed by many perceptive people and for quite some time. Among others, I shall cite below the words of Philip Rieff (1966, p. 57), who related the birth of psychoanalysis to the present age: 'Psychoanalysis is yet another method of learning how to endure the loneliness produced by culture. A tolerance of ambiguities is the key to what Freud considered the most difficult of all personal accomplishments: a genuinely stable character in an unstable time.' The thought expressed in these lines is somewhat similar in sentiment to what I tried to convey in the previously quoted passage from one of my papers. At any rate, what is interesting is the fact that psychoanalysis itself, apart from its being an explorative and individualistic endeavor, seems to have had a supportive function from its very beginning.

CONCLUSION

Juris G. Draguns (1981) notes in his paper, 'Counseling Across Cultures: Common Themes and Distinct Approaches', that contributions from the psychodynamic schools to cross-cultural counseling are lacking. Draguns (1981, p.16) states: 'What is the relevance for the delivery and implementation of cross-cultural counseling services of this theoretical perspective, especially of its emphasis upon intra-psychic conflict and unconscious determinants of behavior?' I think this chapter can be said to be an attempt to meet his challenge. I have tried to offer a theoretical model that can encompass all forms of psychotherapy, and I have indicated that the kind of psychopathology that becomes the object of psychotherapy invariably involves cultural values insofar as they engender psychic conflicts. I have shown that the development of modern psychotherapy in the West manifests this point.

The lesson from the above analysis is obvious. We hear often nowadays that Western psychotherapies cannot be applied to non-Western patients. It is no wonder, because Western psychotherapies presuppose the existence of cultural conflicts peculiar to Western people. As a matter of fact, even in the West the forms of psychotherapy are changing precisely because the cultural conflicts underlying psychic pathology are changing. Thus it is a known fact that the number of patients to whom the classical technique of orthodox psychoanalysis is applicable is decreasing, hence the explosion of new forms of psychotherapy in recent years. But non-Western societies are no less subject to cultural changes, particularly as a result of the thrust of Westernization. This naturally leads to cultural conflicts and thereby makes people susceptible to psychopathology, which requires the application of psychotherapeutic procedures. It is important to remember, however, that the purpose of psychotherapy in non-Western societies is not to promote Westernization; rather, it concerns the conflicts created by Westernization, but it is not the same as promoting Westernization. Psychotherapy tries to aid an otherwise failing traditional identity and strives to reintegrate, when possible, traditional values and imported ones. That is the essence of what we learn from the development of modern psychotherapies in the West.

REFERENCES

Bowlby, J (1971). *Attachment*. London: Penguin.
Burton-Bradley, B. G. (1975). *Stone age crisis: A psychiatric appraisal*. Nashville: Vanderbilt University Press.
Doi, T. (1962). *Amae*: A key concept for understanding Japanese personality structure. In R. J. Smith & R. K. Beardsley (Eds.), *Japanese culture: Its development and characteristics* (pp. 132-139). Chicago: Aldine.
Doi, T. (1963). Some thoughts on helplessness and the desire to be loved. *Psychiatry: Journal for the Study of Interpersonal Processes*, 26, 266-272.
Doi, T. (1964). Psychoanalytic therapy and Western man. A Japanese view. *International Journal of Social Psychiatry*, *I* 13-18.
Doi, T. (1973a). *The anatomy of dependence* (J. Bester, Trans.). Tokyo: Kodansha.
Doi, T. (1973b). Psychotherapy as 'hide and seek'. *Bulletin of the Meninger Clinic*, 37, 174-177.
Draguns, J. G. (1981). Counseling across cultures: Common themes and distinct approaches. In P. Pedersen, J. G. Draguns. W. J. Lonner, & J. E. Trimble (Eds.), *Counseling across cultures*. Honolulu: University Press of Hawaii.
Ellenberger, H. F. (1982). Evolution of the ideas about the nature of the psychotherapeutic process in the Western world. In T. Ogawa (Ed.), *The history of psychiatry: Mental illness and its treatments* (pp. 1-26). Tokyo: Saiko.
Freud, S. (1963). Introductory lectures of psychoanalysis. In *The standard edition of the complete psychological works of Sigmund Freud* (Vol. 16, p. 451). London: Hogarth.
Hartmann, H. (1958). *Ego psychology and the problem of adaptation*. New York: International Universities Press.
Havens, L. L. (1981). Twentieth century psychiatry: A view from the sea. *American Journal of Psychiatry*, *138*, 1279-1287.
Hippler, A. E. (1976). Shamans, curers and personality: Suggestions toward a theoretical model. In W. P. Lebra (Ed.), *Mental health research in Asia and the Pacific: Vol. 4, Culture-bound syndromes, ethnopsychiatry and alternate therapies*. Honolulu: University Press of Hawaii.
Karasu, T. B. (1977). Psychotherapies: An overview. *American Journal of Psychiatry*, *134*, 851-863.
Kondo, K. (1976). The origin of Morita therapy. In W. P. Lebra (Ed.), *Mental health research in Asia and the Pacific: Vol. 4. Culture-bound syndromes, ethnopsychiatry and alternate therapies*. Honolulu: University Press of Hawaii.
Lebra, W. P. (Ed.). (1976). *Mental health research in Asia and the Pacific: Vol. 4. Culture-bound syndromes, ethnopsychiatry and alternate therapies*. Honolulu: University Press of Hawaii.
Marsella, A. J., Tharp, R., & Cibrowski, T. (Eds.). (1979). *Perspectives on cross-cultural psychology*. New York: Academic.
Murase, T. (1976). Naikan therapy. In W. P. Lebra (Ed.), *Mental health research in Asia and*

the Pacific. Vol. 4. Culture-bound syndromes, ethnopsychiatry and alternate therapies. Honolulu: University Press of Hawaii.

Neil, J. R., & Ludwig. A. M. (1980). Psychiatry and psychotherapy: Past and future. American Journal of Psychotherapy, 24, 39-50.

Pedersen, P. B., Draguns, J. G., Lonner, W. J., & Trimble, J. E. (Eds.). (1981). Counseling across cultures. Honolulu: University Press of Hawaii.

Prince, R. (1979). Variations in psychotherapeutic procedures. In A. J. Marsella, R. Tharp, & T. Cibrowski (Eds.), Perspectives on cross-cultural psychology. New York: Academic.

Rieff, P. (1966). The triumph of the therapeutic: Uses of faith after Freud. New York: Harper & Row.

Stone, L. (1961). The psychoanalytic situation. New York: International Universities Press.

van den Berg, J. H. (1974). Divided existence and complex society. Pittsburgh: Duquesne University Press.

Winnicott, D. W. (1965). The maturational process and the facilitating environment. London: Hogarth.

Review of Mamoru Iga, *The Thorn in the Chrysanthemum: Suicide and Economic Success in Modern Japan* (University of California Press, 1986), first published in *Journal of Japanese Studies.* 1987

⑰ The Thorn in the Chrysanthemum: Suicide and Economic Success in Modern Japan

The Thorn in the Chrysanthemum focuses on two outstanding facts of modern Japan, suicide and economic success, with the author assuming a possible connection between the two. In fact, he states in the introductory chapter that the real determinants of Japanese suicide and economic success are value orientations, which he describes in detail in the later chapters. However, his idea of Japanese value orientations is revealed in the preface, as he characterizes modern Japan as a society in transition from feudalism and oligarchy to democracy. He mentions in passing some critical reviews written recently by foreign observers about Japanese culture, emphasizing that his own book will purportedly present a balanced view. But I wonder how balanced it actually is – I can't help feeling after reading it that the chrysanthemum was almost completely choked by the thorn, if not eaten up by worms.

The author mentions twice that there is a sign of revival of traditionalism in Japan with the recent decline of American prestige (pp. 57, 115). He is no doubt right. I also do not deny that it is very important to pinpoint the shortcomings of Japanese culture and society. I do object, however, to his seemingly wholesale condemnation of Japanese culture and society as feudalistic, authoritarian, and monistic. It is not that his condemnation has no substance, but those terms are used too loosely and without definition. I also cannot accept his underlying assumption that history necessarily advances from uncivilized feudalism to enlightened democracy. Furthermore, I am particularly unhappy with his attributing the motivations of suicide directly to those tendencies in Japanese society he singles out. I am not saying that suicide is not related to social conditions, but can Japanese suicides be solely accounted for by those tendencies? If so, how can one explain the fact that even those reared in the land of democracy commit suicide? Perhaps one would argue according to Durkheim that Japanese suicide is altruistic and fatalistic, while American suicide is egoistic and anomic. But surely there must be something common in all suicides irrespective of nationality. Isn't suicide committed in despair, whether altruistic or egoistic, whether Japanese or American? Despair is not a Japanese monopoly, though the author seems to make out that Japanese youth are particularly susceptible to that emotion (p. 23).

I wonder if Iga is familiar with the recent research done by Dr. Kazuya Yoshimatsu's team at the Psychiatric Research Institute of Tokyo which studied the cohort of those born around 1930 and thereafter. Their suicide rate was consistently high in comparison with other cohorts both when they were young, immediately following the defeat in last war, and also in recent years when they passed the age of 50. In fact it was this cohort that gave the impression that Japanese youth had a special attraction to suicide, for the suicide rate of Japanese youth has shown a considerable decrease since then.

The only plausible explanation for the high suicide rate for this particular cohort is that the younger generation naturally suffered most from the social upheaval caused by the defeat in the last war, thus being made vulnerable to subsequent stress. In other words, it is truer to say that the cultural conflict engendered by a social cataclysm, rather than what is conceived vaguely as feudalism or 'authoritarian familism', is responsible for the increased suicide rate. I think this explanation fits in very well with the seemingly curious fact the author points out, namely, that those cities with strong traditional ties show a higher suicide rate in comparison with Metropolitan Tokyo; it is in those cities that the cultural conflict must be more keenly felt. Also, this explanation applies well to the recent increase in the suicide rate of American youth, since it certainly reflects the social and cultural turmoil the United States has undergone in the years following the Vietnam War.

There are a few minor points I would like to raise with regard to the author's use of Japanese terms such as *amae*, *tatemae*, and *honne*. These are everyday words and surely he is entitled to use them as he pleases. However, since he quotes me on *amae*, I have to say that I do not completely agree with his entirely negative interpretation of *amae*. He mentions that *amae* has something to do with status difference. This is true, but what concerns *amae* is a psychological status called dependence. Dependence itself has a bad connotation in English and will usually be equated with inferior social status. Yet not infrequently those of higher social status do indulge in *amae* toward those of lower status without acknowledging the fact. This can be observed whether in Japan or the United States. At any rate, it is simply not true to say that '*amae* itself is possible because of the obsessive concern with status difference' (p. 38). *Amae* primarily refers to a content state of mind when one's need for love is reciprocated by another's love, which begins in infancy. Therefore, one should rather reverse the above statement to the effect that the Japanese preoccupation with status difference was born and maintained precisely because they cherish the primitive feeling of *amae* and want to reproduce it whenever possible. I do not object to his comment about a core element of narcissism being *amae*, but I must point out that the term narcissism, just like *amae*, has been much abused recently (p. 96). There is healthy and morbid narcissism, just as there is adaptive and maladaptive *amae*, a distinction that entirely escapes the author's attention, as he only emphasizes the negative aspect.

I understand why Iga deplores the notorious *tatemae-honne* discrepancy (pp. 19-82, 85, 135, 194). I regret that I cannot go into detail on this subject here, as it has intrigued me for years, so much so that I have recently written a book about it.[1] Referring readers to *The Anatomy of Self* for a fuller statement of my position, let me state here only that the *tatemae-honne* duality has a legitimacy of its own, as it is inherent in human nature. In fact it can be found anywhere, though Japanese can be said to be especially sensitive on this issue, as is attested by the existence of those special terms. The extreme *tatemae-honne* discrepancy is the very product of the social and cultural changes brought about by modernization. In other words, it is indicative of the cultural conflict I mentioned above with regard to suicide. No wonder people began to talk about it more often in postwar years.

Returning to the author's main argument, I find it hard to swallow comments such as the following: 'In traditional Japan, individuals were role carriers rather than humans' (p. 76). This may be construed as true. But what is wrong with being a role carrier? What is a human if he or she has no role to carry? I also do not subscribe to the author's thesis that the exploitation of insecure employees is an important cause of Japan's economic success (pp. 180, 184). Again he may be right. But, whether secure or insecure, isn't it all relative? If the Japanese employee wants to promote his company's profit, believing that it will benefit him eventually, is this all sheer nonsense? Does that only prove that he is duped by the capitalist? In the same vein, I feel uncomfortable with the author's reprehensible statement that Japanese women's alleged control of the household budget is 'that of custodian, not that of co-owners' (p. 182). He underestimates grossly their ingeniousness and insults their sense of responsibility in the marital relationship. I am objecting not so much to his statement of facts as the undertone. He sounds as if traditional Japan was dark and unhuman. Reading through the book I concluded that he is too Americanized and cannot see his country of origin except through the eyes of Americans.

However, at the very end of the book, the next to the last page, I was startled by a sudden switch from the position the author had taken up to this point. He states: 'Despite these weaknesses, Japanese value orientations offer some suggestions for American people to consider. After all, such dichotomous concepts as nonrationality versus rationality and groupism versus individualism represent the two abstract extremes of human potential. The ideal personality combines them in equilibrium' (p. 203). He then marshals the argument in favor of nonrationality, group goals, and authority. All this perhaps does not come to much as it amounts to only about 200 words and is printed in small type. The book ends there abruptly, with no further explanation, no attempt at integration with the rest of the book. This addition seems to be a note reflecting an afterthought.

After pondering the book's puzzling end, I recalled a comment in the middle of the book, that is, 'the Japanese propensity toward the juxtaposition of contradictory ideas without an attempt at logical and ideological integration' (p. 57). The author himself seems to exemplify this propensity in the way he ends the book. I am happy indeed that he has retained one Japanese trait. I hope I am not belittling him in saying this, because it is certainly part of ancient Japanese wisdom to sustain contradictory ideas, if each is viable, without forcing their premature integration. The *tatemae-honne* duality especially well cultivated in Japanese culture also might stem from this primordial tendency in the final analysis. With this reminder, I shall end my review just as abruptly as Iga does his book.

NOTES

1. Takeo Doi, *The Anatomy of Self: The Individual Versus Society* (New York: Kodansha, 1986).

First published in *The International Review of Psycho-Analysis*, Vol.16, Part 3, 1989.
Routledge for The Institute of Psycho-Analysis, London, 1989

⑱ The Concept of *Amae* and its Psychoanalytic Implications

You may wonder why I am introducing a concept which derives from an everyday Japanese word called *amae*. The reason is twofold. First, the concept of *amae* is important as an organizing principle in understanding the emotional life of Japanese people. Second, in spite of its being Japanese in origin it sheds light on and unifies many psychoanalytic concepts that are usually considered separately.

I stumbled, so to speak, on the concept of *amae* in treating Japanese patients psychoanalytically, for I was struck by the fact that their relationship to the therapist is tinged with the same emotional tone which pervades all interpersonal relationships in Japan, the quality that can best be described by a Japanese word *amae*. This is a noun which derives from *amaeru*, an intransitive verb meaning 'to depend and presume upon another's love or bask in another's indulgence'. It has the same root as the word, *amai*, an adjective meaning 'sweet'. Thus *amae* can suggest something sweet and desirable. There exists also a rich vocabulary in the Japanese language centring around the theme of *amae* expressing various phases of its related psychology, a further fact which corroborates the importance of *amae* in the emotional life of the Japanese people. In this respect one can very well say that the concept of *amae* illustrates the characteristics of Japanese people. It has been my belief at the same time that this concept has a universal applicability inasmuch as the patient's transference can be interpreted in terms of *amae*. In other words, the concept of *amae* can lend itself to psychoanalytic formulation and may even complement the existing theories of psychoanalysis. Thus I have written extensively using this concept, both in Japanese and English, and some of my writings might have caught your attention. But so far I have not presented my ideas at an official meeting of the International Psychoanalytical Association and I am very pleased to be given this opportunity to read a paper at this Congress.

In this paper I shall attempt specifically to elucidate the psychoanalytic implications of the concept of *amae*, but before I do so I shall have to describe the usage of the vocabulary of *amae* so that I can acquaint you with the psychology it implies. What is perhaps most important is that it definitely links with the psychology of infancy, because we say about a small child that it is *amaeru*-ing only when it begins to become aware of its surroundings and to seek its mother. Please note that in this instance *amae* describes certain forms of behaviour of the child that directly refers to the feelings revealed by that behaviour. *Amae* can be used not only for a child *vis-à-vis* his mother or any caring person, but also when similar feelings occur in any other interpersonal relationship such as between lovers, friends, husband and wife, teacher and student, employer and employee. Also, please note that one who does *amaeru* on another depends on him or her psychologically since one needs him or her for its fulfilment. However, this does not mean that one who does *amaeru* is necessarily inferior or subordinate in social status to another. In fact it not infrequently happens that one who does *amaeru* is higher in social status, such as the parent depending psychologically on the child or the employer on the employee. However, one who is higher in social status usually either is not aware of his own *amae* on his subordinate or does not wish to admit it openly.

Another important thing about the concept of *amae* is that though it primarily indicates a content state of mind when one's need for love is reciprocated by another's love, it may also refer to that very need for love because one cannot always count on another's love, much as one would wish to do so. Hence it follows that the state of frustration in *amae*, the various phases of which can be described by a number of Japanese words, may also be referred to as *amae* and in fact it often is so called, since obviously *amae* is more keenly felt as a desire in frustration than in fulfilment. It is related to this usage that we can talk of two kinds of *amae*, a primitive one which is sure of a willing recipient and a convoluted one which is not sure if there is such a recipient. The former kind is childlike, innocent and restful: the latter is childish, wilful and demanding: to put it simply, good and bad *amae*, so to speak. This distinction is meaningful psychoanalytically and I shall come back to this later.

From what has been said above one may argue that *amae* is a kind of love. This is surely correct. However, what distinguishes *amae* from the ordinary meanings of love is that it presupposes a passive stance toward one's partner, as it invariably involves a dependence on the receptive partner for its fulfilment, though it is quite possible to pursue such a passive stance actively. Things are rather different with love, as one is supposedly on one's own in loving, even though it too needs a willing recipient if it is to get any pleasure out of loving. The difference between love and *amae* can best be seen in the way these two words are used respectively. You can easily say 'I love you' in order to convey your feeling to whoever you happen to love. Actually the expression is often meant to strike the chord in your partner so that he or she will respond in kind. In fact it seems to me that there is a belief in Occidental countries that love should be expressed in word and deed if it is genuine. But in case of *amae*, you cannot say 'I *amaeru* on you' unless you happen to be in a reflective mood to acknowledge your *amae* on the partner. The point is that the genuine feeling of *amae* should be conveyed and appreciated only non-verbally. In case the wish to *amaeru* is to be literally verbalized, it sounds terribly affected and grossly ingratiating. In other words, verbalization spoils the wish to *amaeru* and makes its true satisfaction virtually impossible.

So much about the usage of *amae* in Japanese and its psychology. Now what is most interesting is that the concept of *amae* suggests a continuous spectrum from early infancy to adulthood. In other words, it agrees with object relations theory and makes it more amenable to introspection precisely because *amae* and its vocabulary refer to inner experience. For instance, passive object love or primary love as defined by Michael Balint can be equated with *amae* in its pure form and as such his concept becomes something quite tangible. In fact Balint deplores the inadequacy of the word 'love' to catch its essence in nascency, and states as follows: 'All European languages are so poor that they cannot distinguish between the two kinds of object-love, active and passive' (1965, p. 56). It is then remarkable that the Japanese language has this word *amae*, enabling the infantile origin of love to be accessible to consciousness. Incidentally I began to correspond with Balint in 1962 and he confirmed, after reading some of my papers, that his ideas and mine were developing in the same direction. I also had the good fortune to discuss the matter with him personally when I went to London in 1964. I was furthermore delighted that he honoured me later by citing my work in his last book, *The Basic Fault*.

In this connexion I would like to say a few words about the concept of attachment, which was introduced by John Bowlby into psychoanalysis from ethology, since it obviously covers the same area as *amae*. As is known, Bowlby sharply distinguishes attachment from dependence, saying that a child does not become attached to his mother because he has to depend on her. So he prefers attachment to dependence as a term, as the former can be more precise than the latter in describing behaviour. He also mentions the negative value implications of the word dependence as another reason for avoiding it. Even so, it seems to me that he overlooks the fact that attachment involves a dependence of its own, as one necessarily becomes dependent on the object as far as one is attached to it. In this regard *amae* definitely has an advantage over attachment precisely because it implies a psychological dependence in the sense mentioned above and unlike attachment refers to the feeling experienced rather than to behaviour. All in all one can say, paradoxical as it may sound, that the concept of *amae* makes it possible to discuss what is not verbalized in ordinary communication, hence is something that remains totally unnoticed if you are speaking European languages.

Next I would like to explain how the concept of *amae* can be related to narcissism, identification and ambivalence. *Amae* is object-relational from the beginning, therefore it does not quite agree with the concept of primary narcissism. However, it fits in very well with secondary narcissism, in fact it is particularly well-suited to describe whatever state of mind may be called narcissistic. Namely, of the two kinds of *amae*, primitive and convoluted, that I mentioned before, the convoluted *amae*, which is childish, wilful and demanding, is surely narcissistic. As a matter of fact, if you suspect someone of being narcissistic, you may be sure that this person has a problem with *amae*. In the same vein, a new concept of self-object defined by Kohut as 'those archaic objects cathected with narcissistic libido' (1971, p. 3) will be much easier to comprehend in the light of *amae* psychology, since 'the narcissistic libido' is none other than convoluted *amae*. Also, Balint's observation that 'in the final phase of the treatment patients begin to give expression to long-forgotten, infantile, instinctual wishes, and to demand their gratification from their environment' (1965, p. 181) makes perfect sense, because the primitive *amae* will manifest itself only after narcissistic defences are worked through by analysis.

As to identification, it is not equivalent to *amae*, rather one should assume that identification develops when *amae* is not satisfied. However, I think Freud, in a roundabout way, comes to recognition of *amae* when he states that 'identification is the original form of emotional tie with an object' (1921, p. 107). For it seems to me that here identification is almost equated with *amae*, since *amae* can be said to be a movement to merge with an object emotionally. Freud mentions elsewhere the affectionate current which constitutes a normal attitude in love along with the sensual current that as the older of the two 'it springs from the earliest years of childhood' (1912, p. 180). Curiously, he did not put together these two statements about identification and affectionate current. Perhaps he couldn't do so without the concept of *amae*. Now it should be quite understandable that *amae* and ambivalence are quite closely related, because *amae* is vulnerable as it totally hinges upon another person for its satisfaction. Hence, it can turn to its opposite at a moment's notice, so to speak. In fact one may say that *amae* is ambivalent from the beginning, just as Freud said about identification (1921, p. 105). In this connexion it would not be out of place to discuss projective identification. It is noteworthy that the recipient of such a projection feels disgusted and disgruntled by the 'pressure via the interpersonal interaction', as Ogden describes it (1979, p. 358). I think such a pull or control by the projector will make sense if it is understood as a form of morbid *amae* on the part of the projector, that is, sweet turned bitter. However, I am not saying that projective identification thus interpreted will be resolved automatically. I should say only that the sensitivity to *amae* will make it easier to detect projective identification when it occurs.

I shall now turn to the question of therapy in terms of *amae*. I think it is safe to assume that whatever conscious motive induces the patient to seek psychoanalytic treatment, the most underlying unconscious motive is that of *amae* or its derivatives. I am not saying that the analyst has to focus on it from the beginning. Nor is it necessary to meet it halfway, that is to say, to respond to it by way of satisfying it. What is important is to keep in mind that it is there, and to wait on it so that it can fully develop in due time in the therapeutic relationship, because I think this is what becomes the kernel of transference. In order to illustrate some of the points I shall use Freud's celebrated case of Dora, 'Fragment of an analysis of a case of hysteria' (1905). It is certainly fragmentary, as the transference did not develop fully there. Or if there was any indication of it, Freud failed to recognize it. But it was precisely in this case study that Freud emphasized the importance of transference for the first time if only to do so by postmortem, so to speak. In other words, this case serves well the purpose of illustrating the importance of transference, and I would also add, the psychology of *amae* in spite of its not being so called by its name. I shall explain this point below. But let me first present a brief outline of the case.

Dora, an 18-year-old intelligent girl of independent spirit, was taken by her father to Freud for treatment. She was attached to her father, but did not get along with her mother at all, whose only hobby was said to be cleaning the house. Dora's family made the acquaintance of a married couple called K in a resort town to which they moved because of her father's illness. Her father then became unusually close to Frau K and Dora too became fond of this lady, visiting K's home frequently to look after their children. Two years before Dora came to treatment, however, she created quite a commotion by accusing Herr K of making advances to her. He vehemently denied the charge claiming that all this was but the figment of her imagination, as she apparently had read some inflammatory books, according to information from his wife. Since then Dora began to ask her father to sever his relation with Frau K, which he refused, while Dora's condition got worse. One day her parents found a suicide note on her desk and following this incident she was brought to Freud for treatment.

I think it is clear that Dora was victimized by those adults around her, a fact which Freud did not deny. But in his treatment he focused upon the role she herself had played in her breakdown. Namely, he tried to make her see that she was secretly in love with Herr K, since she did enjoy his company before, so much so that she knowingly overlooked her father's affair with Frau K. In order to bring this point home to her Freud used dream interpretation exclusively, but after three months of intensive work Dora abruptly announced one day her intention to terminate the treatment on that particular day, which she actually did. She returned to Freud, however, fifteen months later, asking for help because of a minor symptom. He learned from her that she had confronted Herr and Frau K in the meanwhile, forcing an admission from both respectively: that Herr K lied to her father about the advances he made to her, that Frau K did have a love affair with her father. Obviously she thus avenged herself upon them.

Freud then realized that her abrupt termination of the past treatment had been a kind of revenge in displacement, that she must have returned to him this time because of a guilt feeling over the past termination. He felt, however, that he had nothing to offer her at that point and dismissed her by saying that he would 'forgive her for having deprived [him] of the satisfaction of affording her a far more radical cure for her troubles' (1905, p. 122).

Besides the main points of analysis by Freud which I have sketched above, there is one more important element in Dora's case. That is her once genuine attachment to Frau K which Freud discusses as follows in a footnote added a few years later after completion of the text: 'The longer the interval of time that separates me from the end of this analysis, the more probable it seems to me that the fault in my technique lay in this omission: I failed to discover in time and to inform the patient that her homosexual love for Frau K was the strongest unconscious current in her mental life' (1905, p. 120). It was not that Freud was not aware at all of Dora's deep affection for Frau K. He definitely was and even mentioned it at some length in the text. What he missed at the beginning was the extent of the significance it had for her, and naturally he could not recognize it in the transference either. In other words, if we follow this line of reasoning, Dora must have terminated the treatment with Freud because she felt her own person was not appreciated by him, just as it was not appreciated by Frau K. Remember in this regard that Frau K had abandoned Dora for the sake of her own love for Dora's father, thus informing her husband of Dora's reading of inflammatory books. Then, if Freud understood her termination of the treatment in the above-mentioned sense, he would not have spurned her request at a later data to resume treatment. It seems to me that his rejection of her request was almost like revenge on his part for having been deprived of the satisfaction of completing her analysis to its logical end. It looks as if he acted like 'an eye for an eye, a tooth for a tooth'. Only if he had known the depth of Dora's disappointment with Frau K, he would have seen how depressed she was and that she was feeling futile in spite of having revenged herself on Herr and Frau K. Furthermore, Freud would not have invited her revenge on himself in the first place in the form of abrupt termination of the treatment. Rather he could have discerned in her disappointment with Frau K the trace of an even deeper dissatisfaction with her own mother.

I think you may have understood by this time that I am equating what Freud meant by the term 'homosexual love' with *amae*. Namely, I suggest that Dora's attachment to Frau K and her subsequent disappointment can be interpreted in terms of *amae*, though the relationship may well have had an aspect that can be called homosexual. Even so I don't believe that such homosexuality was pathogenic in the case of Dora. Rather it was convoluted *amae* which developed, if it did, into homosexual love under the circumstances. Interestingly, in one of his later papers Freud expresses a similar view to mine with regard to the case of another young girl who was infatuated with a certain 'society lady' to the great dismay of her father. For Freud states that 'the lady-love was a substitute for her mother' (1920, p. 156). Yet lacking a convenient concept like *amae* and also given his theoretical preference, it was inevitable that he gave more weight to the aspect of homosexuality. Thus in the footnote quoted above he introduces the speculation that Dora had a reason to conceal her 'homosexual' love for Frau K, adding as follows: 'Before I had learnt the importance of the homosexual current of feeling in psychoneurotics, I was often brought to a standstill in the treatment of my cases or found myself in complete perplexity' (1905, p. 120).

In concluding this paper I cannot help adding a few more words about what Freud pointed out in the last section of 'Analysis terminable and interminable', since it also can be related to *amae*. I refer to his statement that there are two themes which give a great trouble in analysis, castration anxiety for men and penis envy for women. He then sums up the two by the term 'repudiation of femininity' (1937, p. 252). Now I should say this repudiation of femininity can be interpreted in terms of *amae*, inasmuch as the nature of femininity here implied is something very much like *amae*, an interpretation which I suspect might appeal to Occidentals. At any rate, the repudiation of femininity amounts, in concrete terms, to the rejection of *amae*. It then follows that there is a strong resistance against acceptance of *amae*, if, as I stated above, *amae* constitutes the underlying unconscious motive in seeking psychoanalytic treatment. Only this resistance would take different forms in men and women. For men *amae* can be dangerous, as it spells submission to others. For women *amae* alone is not enough, as they often feel something is missing. I don't know how this proposition sounds to Western psychoanalysts. Does it sound preposterous, just as Freud's original ideas might have sounded preposterous to his contemporaries? But we are only equally human, are we not? Therefore, if something makes sense to us Japanese, it must make sense to you Occidentals as well. Or somebody might raise an objection that I have overemphasized the universality of the concept of *amae*, that I have tried to explain too much by it. Certainly I have related the concept of *amae* to many psychoanalytic concepts that are usually dealt with separately. But it is not that I have simply equated them all. My point is that if the concept of *amae* can be related in a meaningful way to other psychoanalytic concepts usually not related to one another, that fact could only suggest that it can unify them into a more satisfactory theory. I shall be happy indeed if this paper contributed toward this end.

SUMMARY

This paper introduces *amae*, a Japanese concept, because of its special bearing on psychoanalysis. *Amae* primarily describes the behaviour and its accompanying affect of a child seeking his mother or any caring person, but it may refer to the similar situations that occur between adults. *Amae* in its most primitive form is equal to the concept of primary love defined by Michael Balint. It also can be related to the concept of attachment elaborated by John Bowlby and other concepts like narcissism, identification, ambivalence, etc. Freud's case of Dora is cited to illustrate the clinical application of *amae* with a special attention to his notion of homosexual love. The repudiation of femininity, another Freudian notion, is also considered in this regard. It is the author's opinion that the concept of *amae* complements the existing theories or psychoanalysis by unifying many concepts usually not related to one another.

TRANSLATIONS OF SUMMARY

Cet article introduit *amae*, concept japonais, en raison de sa portée particulière en psychoanalyse. *Amae* décrit premièrement le comportement d'un enfant, et l'affect qui l'accompagne, lorsqu'il cherche sa mère ou la personne qui s'occupe de lui, mais ce concept peut renvoyer a des situations analogues qui surviennent entre adultes. *Amae* dans sa forme primitive est equivalent au concept d'amour primaire défini par Michael Balint il peut également être rattaché au concept d'attachement élaboré par John Bowlby et à d'autres concepts comme le narcissisme, l'identification, l'ambivalence, etc. Le cas de Dora de Freud est cité ici pour illustrer l'application clinique d'*amae* et plus particulièrement sa notion de l'amour homosexuel. La répudiation de la féminité, autre notion freudienne, est également envisagée dans ce contexte. Selon l'auteur, le concept d'*amae* complete les théories existantes en psychanalyse en unifiant de nombreux concepts qui ne sont habituellement pas reliés les uns aux autres.

Dieser Beitrag stellt *amae*, ein japanisches Konzept, vor, weil es von besonderer Bedeutung für die Psychoanalyse ist. *Amae* beschreibt in erster Linie das Verhalten und dessen Begleitaffekt eines Kindes, das nach seiner Mutter oder irgendeiner betreuenden Person sucht, es kann sich aber auch auf ähnliche, zwischen Erwachsenen stattfindende Situationen beziehen. *Amae* in seiner primitivsten Form ist dem Konzept der primären Liebe, das von Michael Balint definiert worden ist, gleich. Es kann aber auch mit dem von John Bowlby weiter ausgeführten Konzept von 'Attachment' und anderen Konzepten wie Narzißmus, Identifikation, Ambivalenz, etc. in Verbindung gebracht werden. Freuds Fall Dora wird zur Illustration der klinischen Anwendung von *amae* zitiert, mit besonderer Aufmerksamkeit auf seine Vorstellung von homosexueller Liebe. Die Ablehnung der Weiblichkeit, eine weitere Vorstellung von Freud, wird auch in diesem Zusammenhang betrachtct. Der Meinung des Autors zufolge vervollständigy das Konzept von *amae* die bestehenden psychoanalytischen Theorien durch die Vereinigung von vielen Konzepten, die normalerweise nicht miteinander in Verbindung gebracht werden.

Este articulo introduce el concepto japonés de *amae* por su especial significado para el psicoanálisis. *Amae* describe principalmente la conducta, y el afecto a ésta ligado, de un niño en busca de madre, o de otra persona que lo ame; pero también se puede aplicar a situaciones similares que occurren entre adultos. *Amae* en su forma más primitiva equivale al concepto de amor primario definido por Michael

Balint. Igualmente puede relacionarse con el concepto de apego elaborado por John Bowlby, y con otros conceptos como narcisismo, identificación, ambivalencia, etc. El autor cita el caso de Dora, de Freud, para ilustrar la aplicación clínica de *amae*, prestando espécial atención a su noción de amor homosexual. Considera también bajo esta luz la repudiación de la femininidad, otra noción freudiana. En opinion del autor el concepto de *amae* complementa las teorías psicoanalíticas existentes, al unificar muchos conceptos que normelmente no se relacionan entre sí.

REFERENCES

Balint, M.(1965). *Primary Love and Psycho-Analytic Technique*. New York: Liveright Publishing Corporation.
—— (1968). *The Basic Fault*. London: Tavistock Publications.
Bowlby, J. (1971). *Attachment and Loss*, Volume 1. London: Pelican Books.
Doi, T. (1962). Amae: a key concept for understanding Japanese personality structure. *Japanese Culture*, ed. R. J. Smith & R. K. Beardsley. Chicago: Aldine Publishing.
—— (1963). Some thoughts on helplessness and the desire to be loved. *Psychiatry*, 26: 266-272.
—— (1973). *The Anatomy of Dependence*. Tokyo: Kodansha International.
Freud, S. (1905). Fragment of an analysis of a case of hysteria. *S.E.* 7.
—— (1912). On the universal tendency to debasement in the sphere of love. *S.E.* 11.
—— (1920). The psychogenesis of a case of homosexuality in a woman. *S.E.* 18.
—— (1921). Group psychology and the analysis of the ego. *S.E.* 18.
—— (1937). Analysis terminable and interminable. *S.E.* 23.
Kohut, H. (1971). *The Analysis of the Self*. New York: Int. Univ. Press.
Ogden, T. H. (1979). On projective identification. *Int. J. Psychoanal.*, 60: 357-373.
Wisdom, J. O. (1987). The concept of 'amae'. *Int. Rev. Psychoanal.*, 14: 263-264.

First published in *Distinguished Lecture Series,* Japan Society of New York, 1989

⑲ The Japanese Psyche: Myth and Reality

O ne could question the legitimacy of talking about the Japanese mind. One may say that there is no such thing as the Japanese mind, or if there is, it is not proved yet, for we only know that there exist individuals who are called Japanese. Naturally, there is a great variety among them, and we should not generalize from selected samples. That is the criticism raised by scholars of the empiricist persuasion against the indigenous studies of the Japanese mind, which have become quite popular in recent years. My own work is often mentioned as one example of these indigenous studies. In reply, I say that it is legitimate to talk about the Japanese mind just as it is legitimate to talk about the American mind. There are phenomena which require explanation in terms of the group mind, such as the differences between cultures or the historical development of various nations. I admit that such explanations would be hypothetical or, one might even say, fictive. However, this does not invalidate the explanations, since any explanation about any subject is hypothetical in the last analysis, and the validity of hypothesis hinges upon how much it can explain.

Any discussion of the Japanese mind – or the American mind for that matter – involves value judgement. Consider, for instance, Allan Bloom's now famous *The Closing of the American Mind*, a severe indictment of cultural decay that seems to be eating away at the American mind today. Along the same line, though totally different in approach, is Christopher Lasch's *The Culture of Narcissism*. Interestingly, there are no such books written by Japanese authors about the Japanese mind. Quite the reverse, almost all recent studies of the Japanese mind seem to emphasize, in positive terms, its unique qualities. Indeed, this tendency is so marked that it has invited some strong reaction, mostly from abroad. Peter N. Dale's *The Myth of Japanese Uniqueness* is a particularly caustic criticism of Japanese uniqueness, which relies solely on an ideological interpretation of history to erroneously conclude that these studies are the products of a nationalistic fervor.

Perhaps it is altogether unwise to use the word 'unique' in describing the different qualities of the Japanese mind, because it might appear that we are implying that the Japanese mind is unrivaled and beyond comparison. If so, this would call to memory the xenophobic nationalism that swept through prewar and wartime Japan. The term unique may even seem offensive when the 'uniqueness of the Japanese' is proposed as an explanation of Japan's remarkable transition from a completely shattered nation to a great world power in mere decades. This smacks of ethnocentrism and such an ethnocentrism, whether of the West or of Japan, is wholly unacceptable. So let us be clear that if the Japanese mind is unique, it is only in the sense that any nation or any person is unique.

One should not suppose, however, that there is nothing in common, say, between the Japanese mind and the American mind. We are all human first and foremost. There are more traits in common that bind us than there are differences that separate us from one another. In other words, I don't subscribe to cultural relativism as such, which dictates that any culture should be judged only on its own terms, that it cannot and should not be tampered with, and that it should not be criticized from the outside. It seems to me that cultural relativism and ethnocentrism are two sides of the same coin. Indeed, why should I be talking to you about the Japanese mind if it concerns us Japanese alone? I am not presenting the Japanese mind as a curiosity, as something beyond your comprehension, and certainly not as an enigma. I present the Japanese mind as food for thought, just as the American mind has been food for Japanese thought for many years.

Some of you might think that I am much too cautious. Yet, this cautious attitude of mine exemplifies one psychological trait which is quite common among Japanese people. If I were American, I would probably have opened my talk with a humorous anecdote to put you at ease. I would have disarmed you at the beginning with a laugh; I would have exuded confidence by presenting myself as attractive and interesting right from the beginning. That tactic, however, is not generally available to us Japanese; it is reserved for a professional comic storyteller called a *rakugo-ka*. Our common philosophy is that one should present oneself as modest, as one who depends entirely upon the goodwill of others. This dependent posture is very important in relating to people in Japan. I am not saying that Japanese are more dependent than Americans. We are equally dependent; however, it is the emphasis on dependence that distinguishes Japanese from Americans and is a prominent feature of the Japanese mind.

When I first came to the United States for psychiatric training in 1950, I was immediately struck by the dramatic difference between the way people in Japan relate to one another and the way Americans relate to one another. I realized that the difference lies in the tolerance for dependent relationships in Japan and the lack of this tolerance in the United States. This observation, it seems to me, is borne out by the existence of a special vocabulary in Japanese to express various phases of emotional dependence. While I do not want to go into details of the language, it should be noted that the word *amae* plays a pivotal role in the lexicon of dependent relationships. *Amae* refers primarily to infant psychology in that it indicates what an infant feels toward its mother when it wants to come close to her and be accepted by her. From this observation, I have concluded that the dependent relationships the Japanese seem to enjoy must be an extension of one's original dependency toward one's parents. It can be further concluded that it is possible to study child-rearing in light of *amae*.

Actually, this idea was put into practice by my friend, the late Dr. William Caudill, cultural anthropologist and pioneer in a cross-cultural study of Japan and the United States. He and his assistant, Mrs. Helen Weinstein, selected a matched sample of thirty three-to-four month-old Japanese and American infants and studied the interactions of those infants with their mothers. The conclusion they drew from this study is extremely interesting:

> American infants are more happily vocal, more active and more exploratory of their bodies and their physical environment than are Japanese infants. Directly related to these findings, the American mother is in greater vocal interaction with her infant and stimulates him to greater physical activity and exploration. The Japanese mother, in contrast, is in greater bodily contact with her infant and soothes him toward physical quiescence and passivity with regard to his environment. Moreover, these patterns of behavior, so early learned by the infant, are in line with the differing expectations for late behavior in the two cultures as the child grows to be an adult.

This observation is highly descriptive of the differences between American and Japanese patterns of communication. Americans are conditioned from the very beginning of life to associate human contact with verbal communication, whereas Japanese tend to emphasize non-verbal communication in everyday transactions. This characteristic of Japanese people, in my view, is related to the psychology of *amae*. In an interaction between the mother and child, the mother of course, can verbalize her feelings, but the infant naturally cannot.

By naming that nonverbal feeling *amae* and also supplying other words for other feelings related to *amae*, the Japanese demonstrate their appreciation of what ordinarily passes unspoken in everyday communication. There is, however, one important distinction about the vocabulary of *amae*: the words describe an emotion but in themselves are not emotive as the English word 'love' is. One could even say that, for Japanese, verbal communication is something that accompanies and supplements non-verbal communication and not the other way around. Perhaps that is why the Japanese often impress foreigners as not properly communicative, not so open and forthright as they should be, if judged by American standards. This comes about because Japanese are extremely sensitive to the feelings surrounding interpersonal relationships and tend to neglect verbal communication.

Apropos of what has been discussed, one might note an interesting difference between what Japanese and Americans understand by 'close relationship'. Japanese feel that with a close friend or lover or spouse one does not have to say much; they are happy simply being together and will not waste time in just talking. In fact, one way the Japanese characterize a close relationship is that they can be comfortably silent together. It seems to me that Americans are quite different in this respect: being close to someone means being able to talk with that person to one's heart's content.

Yet Japanese at times do enjoy talking, just as Americans can enjoy moments of silence, perhaps only momentarily. Also, in the same context, you may have noticed the Japanese shyness – reluctance, really – about demonstrating affection in public. Lovers, spouses or parents and children do not embrace or kiss in public, simply because they do not want to make public what should remain private. Only shaking hands among the Western forms of greeting has become somewhat fashionable nowadays – besides traditional bowing – particularly among city people; but this still is done less frequently than in the West. These patterns of social behavior are part of the Japanese propensity for estimating at first meeting how much they can or should be dependent and deferential toward one another. (Again the *amae* factor.)

The preference of Japanese for nonverbal communication within the group is workable only among those who know each other intimately. And what Japanese value most in group life is the sense of belonging. Actually, the very purpose of socialization is to gain this sense of belonging which is inculcated in children from very early infancy on. No wonder, then, that Japanese love group life, which they generally experience as supportive and not as constrictive. Of course, a group can be constrictive; however, the Japanese style of group control is not authoritarian, not really from the top down. The well-known consensus-building proceeds inconspicuously from the bottom up. Also, one must remember that the Japanese identification with a group is never meant to be total: Japanese do experience conflict between individual interests and group life. How to manage such conflict is no small matter to a Japanese.

The importance of the question of how to manage this individual-vs-group conflict of interest is related to the problem of ambivalence, which in the technical parlance of psychiatry means the coexistence of opposite feelings toward the same object. It was Freud who promoted the theory that ambivalence is inherent in human nature. Even though it is accepted that ambivalence is universal, there are individual differences and, I strongly suspect, cultural differences as well in the ways of coping with it. It seems to me that Westerners, and possibly Chinese, tend to put ambivalence out of mind and stress instead a particular strategy in resolving conflict: they try not to reveal the existence of conflict whenever possible.

Japanese, on the contrary, seem to dwell on ambivalence and may at times even appear to be playing with two opposite feelings. This is where the Japanese classical duality of *tatemae* and *honne* comes in. *Tatemae* describes the rules of whatever group one happens to belong to. Japanese observe tatemae – the social obligation – as long as it also contains *honne* – one's personal considerations. But when it no longer does, they feel entitled to act out *honne* – to express the previously unstated interests.

It is this pattern of behavior that is usually interpreted as Japanese unscrupulousness, a Japanese distaste for confrontation or ambiguity. It is this pattern that often gives Westerners the impression that Japanese are being hypocritical and opportunistic. In more neutral terms they can be said to be relativistic and flexible; and of course, depending upon circumstances, this can also be interpreted as a sign of weakness or of shrewdness.

Do these *tatemae/honne* concepts apply to Americans? I think they do, in spite of the appearance that defies such duality. But whichever of the two aspects is adopted, Americans vigorously justify it; the Japanese do not.

I think this attitude of the Japanese very much affects their relationships with foreigners. If they show their ambivalence to each other, they will naturally manifest it even more toward foreigners, in turn inviting foreigners' ambivalence. The upshot of all this is that they may not really be liked by foreigners in spite of an ardent desire to be liked. This, incidentally, explains the rather poor performance by Japanese in international diplomacy. In particular, they do not seem to be able to exert leadership in the arena of international politics. But how can they when they have the same problem in domestic politics? This is the root of the Japanese problem which so vexes Americans.

I would like to say a few words about the function of the Emperor in Japan. The funeral of the Showa Emperor attracted much coverage of this subject on American television. According to the present Constitution, the emperor is the symbol of the unity of Japan as a nation; this definition seems to make sense in the light of what I have said before. There is much division and tension in Japanese society because of the pervasive atmosphere of ambivalence. The emperor is said to unite the nation, not with power, but with his status as the symbol of national unity. He is not even emperor in the true sense of the word, even though Japan waged past imperial wars in his name. He is essentially a tribal chief with an added religious function. In fact, he is totally dependent, like an infant, upon his subordinates. Yet he is accorded the highest rank – an acknowledgement of the dignity of dependence. One might say that this paradox comes from a myth, and I say, surely, it is a living myth. It is widely perceived that Japanese, compared with Westerners, can be naively, sometimes blindly, trusting toward fellow human beings – so much so that the Japanese as a whole are often labeled as too paternalistic for a modern nation, which arouses negative reactions from western critics like Peter Dale (*The Myth of Japanese Uniqueness*). But this is indeed fact, not something fabricated or politically maneuvered into being.

I am not saying that everything has been all right with this myth. The fact is that it was much inflated in prewar and wartime Japan, and the emperor was exploited by the militarists just as the trusting population was abused. Thus, when the emperor became the focus of attention all over the world because of his illness and subsequent death, there arose a renewed interest in his possible culpability as a war criminal. It has been remarked upon that the Japanese, in general, do not seem to talk about their war guilt as much as they should, as Germans do. I think this is true. In fact, I myself would not like to discuss this matter in front of you either. Since it concerns our subject, the Japanese mind, I at least want to add that because Japanese do not want to talk openly about their guilt, it does not mean that they do not feel guilty. I think the Showa Emperor was certainly aware of his culpability and must have felt truly grateful that he was not tried openly. He simply did not wish to let his personal feelings be known. Japanese are simply diffident, or inhibited, about this matter of guilt; you might say that it also could be an expression of ambivalence. Certainly it exemplifies their distaste for confrontation. Whether good or bad, this is the Japanese mind.

Japanese talking about their guilt openly and unabashedly! I do not know if it will change in the foreseeable future or if it should change. I, for one, hope that I shall not live to see it. With this hope – that the soul of Japan will not change – I close this lecture.

First published in James W. Stigler, Richard A. Shweder, Golbert Herdt (Eds), *Cultural Psychology: Essays on Comparative Human Development*, Cambridge University Press, 1990

⑳ The Cultural Assumptions of Psychoanalysis

I have decided to use as a point of departure for this discussion a quotation from Freud that clearly indicates that he was aware of the cultural context in which psychoanalysis was born and is practiced. In discussing the cross-cultural insights into psychoanalysis, I consider Freud's ideas first because psychoanalysis is, after all, his brainchild. Surely there is nowadays increasing diversity in psychoanalytic theory and practice, but Freud is 'still our lost object, our unreachable genius, whose passing we have never properly mourned', the 'father who doesn't die', as Dr. Wallerstein aptly put it in his presidential address, 'One Psychoanalysis or Many', at the 1987 International Congress of Psychoanalysis. In plain language, one might just as well say that the ghost of Freud is still uniting the entire body of psychoanalysts, if not hovering over them. Perhaps this is as it should be, but I feel there is something in Dr. Wallerstein's remark that deserves our further consideration, and I shall come back to it at the end of this chapter. At any rate, I discuss psychoanalysis only to the extent that it is still dominated by Freud's original thinking.

Now the quotation from Freud that I want to use is in his essay, 'The Future Prospects of Psychoanalytic Therapy'. As its title suggests, the paper has an exuberant tone, promising a substantial improvement in therapeutic prospects of psychoanalysis. According to Freud's reasoning, the improvement will come from three directions: advances in knowledge and technique, increased authority of the psychoanalyst, and the general effect of psychoanalytic enlightenment of the general population. What I would like to quote is the beginning of the paragraph that introduces the discussion of increased authority of the psychoanalyst:

> I have said that we had much to expect from the increase in authority which must accrue to us as time goes on. I need not say much to you about the importance of authority. Only very few civilized people are capable of existing without reliance on others or are even capable of coming to an independent opinion. You cannot exaggerate the intensity of people's inner lack of resolution and craving for authority. The extraordinary increase in neuroses since the power of religions has waned may give you a measure of it. (1910b: 146)

This passage is interesting on several points. First of all, Freud is surprisingly forceful in acknowledging the necessity of authority for human beings. In fact his statement is made in such general terms that it could refer even to himself or other like-minded people who otherwise would not deign to depend on others. Implicit here is his recognition that the authority is there primarily to sustain people. In other words, there seems to be a reciprocity between the exercise of authority and the people's need. Again noteworthy is his suggestion that the contemporary increase in neuroses is related to the decline of authority of religion. Would it not follow then that if psychoanalysis purports to cure neuroses, it somehow takes the place of religion with regard to authority, even though it won't be just a substitute for religion? At any rate, it seems to me that his expectation of increased authority for the future psychoanalyst would be realized only in such a context. That is to say, authority removed from religion would be added to psychoanalysis.

I hope in reasoning like this I am not too far from what Freud actually might have thought of. However, he did not pursue this line, as obviously he did not want psychoanalysis to be associated with religion even remotely. Thus, right after the quoted passage, he changed to a related thought that society was not kindly disposed toward psychoanalysis at the beginning because it was too novel and will never embrace it whole-heartedly because it takes society to task for causing neuroses. Will his expectation of increased authority for the future psychoanalyst come to nothing, then? To this quandary he offers the following consolation: 'And yet the situation is not so hopeless as one might think at the present time. Powerful though men's emotions and self-interest may be, yet intellect is a power too – a power which makes itself felt, not, it is true, immediately, but all the more certainly in the end' (1910b: 147). Now it will be very interesting to examine his reasoning so far. At the beginning he seems to covet authority for psychoanalysis. On second thought, he doubts its feasibility. Then he ends up espousing the cause of pure intellect for psychoanalysis. If that is his reasoning, did he give up the claim to authority for psychoanalysis? He does not say so, leaving the question of authority up in the air for the moment. But when one comes to the very end of this essay, it becomes clear that he really did not let go the claim to authority completely, because he seems to be setting hopes on the turnabout of social authority as a result of the enlightenment of the whole population by psychoanalysis. All in all, will it be too much to say that Freud's attitude toward authority was rather ambiguous, if not clearly ambivalent?

I think this way of thinking sheds a new light on the nature of psychoanalytic therapy as Freud conceived it. For there is reason to believe that not only could Freud not assume authority for the psychoanalyst for the time being, but evidently he even postulated that the psychoanalyst should not play the role of authority in the way religion did for the faithful. True, the psychoanalytic relationship is not symmetrical, since 'it presupposes the consent of the person who is being analyzed and a situation in which there is a superior and a subordinate', as Freud put it (1914:49). But this superior position of analyst does not entail authority in the usual sense of the word as it appears, for instance, in the previously quoted passage from Freud; rather, it corresponds to that of expert, since the main task of the psychoanalyst is to assist the patient in interpreting his mental state. In other words, the analyst is very much task-oriented and will hardly cater to the patient's dependency need. Still, one might protest that the discretion on the part of the analyst will not prevent people from looking up to him as authority, which certainly is the case. But, then, since he is supposed not to nurture and sustain people, his authority would be a very impersonal one, indeed, like that of an efficient bureaucrat. In other words, he would appear even as an authoritarian figure at times. This is exemplified by none other than Freud, and I shall cite his treatment of Dora as an example to explain my point.

First, a brief outline of the case is in order. Dora, an 18-year-old girl, was brought to Freud by her father because of a suicide note she left on her desk. The turn of events that led up to this outcome was rather ugly, to say the least. She was nearly seduced by a friend of her father's, when her father himself was having an affair with the friend's wife. The seducer denied the fact of seduction and she entreated her father to sever the relationship with his friend's wife. But his having refused to comply with her wish finally drove her to suicidal thoughts. Now I don't know if Freud felt sympathy for the poor girl. If he did, it was not recorded. What was recorded is that he worked intensively on her assumed infatuation with the seducer, utilizing thereby dream interpretation extensively. One day, three months after the treatment started, when he expressed satisfaction at the result of dream interpretation, she replied 'in a depreciatory tone': 'Why, has anything so very remarkable come out?' Then at the following session all of a sudden she announced her decision to terminate the treatment on that very day. Freud was not visibly shaken by her unexpected move and said, 'You know that you are free to stop the treatment at any time. But for today we will go on with our work' (1905:105). So the hour was spent as usual. Shouldn't one be amazed by his aloofness? I believe, however, that contrary to his seeming calmness, he was deeply disappointed by the abrupt termination of her treatment. This is borne out by the fact that he explains at some length his afterthoughts of why he did not urge her to stay on in treatment, that is, why he let her go, and, furthermore, by what happened afterward. Namely, when she returned to him 15 months later asking for help because of a minor symptom, he dismissed her, saying that he had nothing to offer her this time and would 'forgive her for having deprived [him] of the satisfaction of affording her a far more radical cure for her troubles' (1905:122). Don't you think that Freud was very authoritarian in all this? My point is that, busy as he was forgiving Dora's alleged offenses, he was totally deaf to her cry for help. I should say, however, that he is not to blame for this, after all, because this would have been inevitable if psychoanalytic therapy consisted in only giving the kind of service an expert could give.

Please don't take me wrong on this matter. I am not saying that Freud always behaved like this toward his patients. On the contrary, he is known to have been very cordial, even collegial, especially if the analysand was someone who wanted to learn from him. But apparently he could have become authoritarian when provoked. And I should think this stems mainly from Freud's ambivalence about taking the role of authority *vis-à-vis* those who crave it. Another example to prove this point can be found in his analysis of religion, as set forth in his essay, 'The Future of an Illusion'. He argues there that religion is an illusion because it is based on wishful thinking and converts helplessness into an unrealistic belief that one is taken care of by a beneficent Providence. Against such an illusion he contrasts the attitude of those who 'admit to themselves the full extent of their helplessness and their insignificance in the machinery of the universe'. He compares their positions to that of 'a child who has left the parental house where he was so warm and comfortable'. Then he insists, 'But surely infantilism is destined to be surmounted' (1927:49). In other words, he disapproves of religion precisely because it serves as authority for those who desperately need help. To this argument of his I would say that the feeling of helplessness is surely attended to in religion, but that it will never be eliminated thereby; if anything, it will be cultivated or even refined, whereas it is more likely to be downgraded or blotted out by psychoanalysis, which presupposes that one should surmount 'infantilism'. No wonder that Freud sounds authoritarian or authoritative, or even pontifical, in explaining away religion in the name of rationality – by so doing he succeeds in brushing aside dependence and helplessness out of his personal view.

I think you can see that I am putting authority and dependence together as a set. That is to say, authority presupposes dependence, just as dependence presupposes authority. Evidently Freud could see that relationship very well, as the above-quoted passage clearly indicates. However, since he was ambivalent about authority, he couldn't tolerate dependence, and thus he ended up being authoritarian. This is my critique of Freud in a nutshell, and formulated like this it would look very simple, almost self-explanatory, as though anybody could have thought it out. However, in my case it was cross-cultural experiences that led me to arrive at this critique. Therefore, I would like to convey the essence of those experiences in the following paragraph.

After I first went abroad to study in the United States, I was immediately struck by the different way that people relate to one another in Japan and the United States, I realized that the difference lies in the tolerance for dependent relationships in Japan and the lack of tolerance in the United States, a fact that is borne out by the existence of a special vocabulary in Japanese to express various phases of emotional dependence. I don't want to go into details on the matter of language here. Suffice to say that the word *amae*, which plays a pivotal role in the vocabulary, originally refers to infant psychology in that it indicates what an infant feels toward its mother when it wants to come close to her and is accepted by her. This observation made me think two things. One, the dependent relationships that the Japanese seem to enjoy are the extension of dependency toward parents. Two, the theme of *amae* is relevant to psychoanalytic theory as it supplies a conceptual tool for developmental psychology. Thus in the light of this insight I came to review the concepts Freud invented to account for infant psychology, especially narcissism and omnipotence. (For more detailed discussion of my view, see Doi, 1962, 1963, 1964, 1969.)

Next, let me quote the pertinent passages from Freud in order to comment on them.

> The primary narcissism of children which we have assumed and which forms one of the postulates of our theories of the libido, is less easy to grasp by direct observation than to confirm by inference from elsewhere. If we look at the attitude of affectionate parents toward their children, we have to recognize that it is a revival and reproduction of their own narcissism, which they have long since abandoned. (1914: 90-91)

> The situation is that of loving oneself, which we regard as the characteristic feature of narcissism. Then, according as the object or the subject is replaced by an extraneous one, what results is the active aim of loving or the passive one of being loved – the latter remaining near to narcissism. (1915:133)

> This extension of the libido theory . . . receives reinforcement . . . from our observations and views on the mental life of children and primitive peoples. In the latter we find characteristics which, if they occurred singly, might be put down to megalomania: an overestimation of the power of their wishes and mental acts, the 'omnipotence of thoughts', a belief in the thaumaturgic force of words – 'magic' – which appears to be a logical application of these grandiose premises. In the children of today, whose development is much more obscure to us, we expect to find an exactly analogous attitude toward the external world. (1914:75)

In the first quotation Freud is clearly begging the question. Because it is much more reasonable to think of the attitude of affectionate parents as a revival and reproduction of their own, still-continuing desire to be loved and cared for, rather than to derive this desire from the hypothetical concept of primary narcissism. The second quotation repeats the same idea as the first in a different form, but there is added an interesting thought that relates the desire to be loved closely to narcissism. I think the expression 'narcissistic gratification', which came to be widely used, originally stems from this idea of Freud's. The third quotation applying the concept of omnipotence to the psychology of children may be descriptive, but I can't help feeling that its description is a bit comical, if not derisive, because actually in all cases of so-called omnipotence of thought the person so described is often fearful, at least objectively quite helpless. Thus one can say that the terms of narcissism and omnipotence actually serve to hide or explain away the bottom fact of human dependence and helplessness.

To do justice to Freud, it is not that he was not cognizant of human dependence and helplessness in infancy. He even noted in his later work that this fact of dependence and helplessness 'establishes the earliest situations of danger and creates the need to be loved' (1926:155). As a matter of fact, I wonder if it would not be too wide of the mark to equate the need to be loved he mentions here with *amae*. But it is true nonetheless that he really wanted to get rid of dependence and helplessness if possible at all, as was manifest in the argument he developed in 'The Future of an Illusion'. In this connection it would be worthwhile to remember that the term 'omnipotence' was primarily used to refer to the Judeo-Christian God. Also, even though the term 'narcissism' was taken from Greek mythology, the concept of loving oneself that it indicates may evoke a godlike quality as it predicates the original state of being as that of complete self-sufficiency. It is then conceivable that Freud could apply with impunity to human psychology the concepts originally reserved for God precisely because the power of religion was waning in Western societies.

You can now see that beginning with the cross-cultural experiences and explaining how they made me reexamine some of the concepts Freud invented I have now come full circle and arrived at the same critique of Freud I set forth first. Namely, his ideas clearly reflect the intellectual climate of Western societies around the turn of the century. In fact, Freud's ambivalence about authority and dependence can be better understood against this background, since both authority and dependence have been closely tied up with Christianity in Western societies. That is to say, if Christianity loses its credibility, both authority and dependence also have to become suspect. Thus Freud felt it necessary to explain them away or else to posit them somehow inside the individual psyche. The result then has been, as we know, a beautiful intellectual construct of libidinal development from primary narcissism onward. The only trouble with this construct, however, is that it tends to be a closed system.

To turn our eyes to the Japanese scene, it of course is entirely different from what prevails in the West. For the world of *amae* is an everyday phenomenon and the Japanese are more likely to be deferential toward authority than not, as they have very few hang-ups about authority. As you know, Japan was never converted to Christianity as a nation, hence cannot be affected by the decline of its influence. In other words, inherent in the Japanese psyche is the polytheistic and animistic ethos and to that extent it is immune from Western secular rationalism. In this connection I would like to mention the question I am often asked by Americans, that is, 'Why is psychoanalysis not popular in Japan?' The usual answer I give to them is as follows. 'Can you tell me why it became popular in the United States? If you can, then I can tell you why it didn't in Japan.' So what I really want to say is that psychoanalysis cannot take root in Japan unless it sheds its cultural bias. But surely it works beautifully with the Japanese if it is prepared to deal with authority and dependence as something truly to be reckoned with. In order to avoid misunderstanding, let me say that I am not suggesting that authority and dependence do not count for the Western patients. They do, as a matter of fact. All I am saying is that there has been a silent conspiracy between psychoanalysis and Western culture in general, at least until recently, in neglecting those issues. But surely this neglect cannot go on forever.

Now in conclusion I will go back to Dr. Wallerstein's remark, as I promised in the beginning. He said in effect that Freud can still function as a rallying point for all divergent schools of psychoanalysis since he is 'our lost object', the 'father who doesn't die'. This appellation of Freud may be a quite appropriate one. But what puzzles me is that it does remind us of Freud's own definition of God. Namely, he stated that 'a personal God is, psychologically, nothing other than an exalted father' (1910a:123). Then, by the same logic, should we think that Freud is a personal God for us psychoanalysts if he is a 'father who doesn't die'? This surely sounds awkward. Or should I perhaps say, God forbid? There is of course no denying that Freud was a great genius. He created a new method of investigation and thus became the founder of psychoanalysis. We learned a great deal from him and shall continue to do so for many days and years to come. But if we take him for 'father who doesn't die', psychoanalysis might become a substitute religion. Then, as such, Freud's remark that 'young people lose their religious belief as soon as their father's authority breaks down' (1910a, p. 123) would come to apply to psychoanalysis as well. In order to make this point clear, let me once more recapitulate what we have discussed so far. According to what Freud stated in the essay I first introduced, the psychoanalyst could not and should not assume authority. But if he comes to identify with Freud as a 'father who doesn't die', is he not assuming authority surreptitiously or simply borrowing Freud's authority? But we have to remember that Freud's authority is not to sustain people, as it does not go beyond that of an expert. In other words, it does not stay put and one knows not when it falls. Therefore, the analyst who rests on Freud's authority is bound to fall when Freud falls. I am afraid that is why contemporary psychoanalysis is losing the advantages it was once thought to possess.

REFERENCES

Doi, T. 1962. *Amae*: A key concept for understanding Japanese personality structure. In Robert J. Smith & Richard K. Beardsley (Eds.), *Japanese culture: Its development and characteristics*. Wenner-Gren Foundation for Anthropological Research.
—— 1963. Some thoughts on helplessness and the desire to be loved. *Psychiatry* 26:266-272.
—— 1964. Psychoanalytic therapy and 'Western man': A Japanese view. *Int. J. Social*

Psychiatry, Special edition, No. 1, 13-18.

—— 1969. Japanese psychology, dependency need and mental health. In W. Caudill & T. Lin (Eds.), *Mental health research in Asia and the Pacific*. Honolulu: East-West Center.

Freud, S. 1905. Fragments of an analysis of a case of hysteria. *Standard edition of the complete works of Sigmund Freud*, vol. 8. London: Hogarth Press, 1953.

—— 1910a. Leonardo da Vinci and a memory of his childhood. *Standard edition of the complete works of Sigmund Freud*, vol. 11. London: Hogarth Press, 1953.

—— 1910b. The future prospects of psychoanalytic therapy. *Standard edition of the complete works of Sigmund Freud*, vol. 11. London: Hogarth Press, 1953.

—— 1914. On narcissism: An introduction. *Standard edition of the complete works of Sigmund Freud*, vol. 14. London: Hogarth Press, 1953.

—— 1915. Instincts and their vicissitudes, *Standard edition of the complete works of Sigmund Freud*, vol. 14. London: Hogarth Press, 1953.

—— 1926. Inhibitions, symptoms and anxiety. *Standard edition of the complete works of Sigmund Freud*, vol. 20. London: Hogarth Press, 1953.

—— 1927. The future of an illusion. *Standard edition of the complete works of Sigmund Freud*, vol. 21. London. Hogarth Press, 1953.

Wallerstein, R. 1987. One psychoanalysis or many. *Int. J. Psycho-Anal.* 69:5-21.

First published in *Infant Mental Health Journal*, Vol.13, No.1, Spring 1992. © Michigan Association for Infant Mental Health

㉑ On the Concept of *Amae*

ABSTRACT: A concept deriving from the Japanese word *amae* is introduced as that which bridges dependence and attachment, two conceptually different states. The word primarily refers to what an infant feels when seeking his or her mother, but it can also apply to an adult to indicate the presence of a similar feeling of being emotionally close to another. Significantly, the feeling of *amae* is not mediated by words, though it can be acknowledged as such on reflection. Also, when frustrated, it can easily lead to a desire for such a feeling. Two popular stories, one French and the other American, are cited to illustrate the existence of *amae*, and, in fact, its central importance, even in non-Japanese contexts. The psychology of keeping pets can also be understood in terms of *amae*. It is thus maintained that though the concept comes from Japanese, it is universally applicable and can shed new light on the emotional life which has been the main target of psychoanalytic investigation.

RÉSUMÉ: Un concept qui dérive du terme japonais *amae* est présenté. L'*amae* relie da dépendance et l'attachement, deux états conceptuellement diffèrents. Ce terme fait avant tout référence à ce que ressent un nourrisson quand il cherche sa mere, mais ii peut aussi s'appliquer à un adulte pour indiquer la présence d'un sentiment similaire, le sentiment d'être émotionnellement proche d'une autre personne. Non sans intérêt, le sentiment d'*amae* n'est pas traduit en mots, même s'il peut être reconnu en tant que tel après réflexion. Lorsque frustré, ii peut également conduire à un désir pour un tel sentiment. Deux histoires populaires, l'une francaise et l'autre americaine, sont citées de façon à illustrer non seulement l'existence de l'*amae*, mais aussi son importance cruciale, même dans des contextes qui ne sont pas japonais. La psychologie qui consiste à avoir des animaux domestiques peut aussi s'expliquer en termes d'*amae*, Nous soutenons donc que, bien que ce concept vienne du japonais, il est universellement applicable et peut éclairer d'une nouvelle façon la vie émotionnelle sur laquelle se sont plus particulièrement penchées les recherches psychanalytiques.

RESUMEN: Un concepto que se deriva de la palabra japonesa *amae* se introduce como aquél que enlaza la dependencia y la unión afectiva, los cuales son dos estados conceptualmente diferentes. La palabra se refiere en principio a lo que el infante siente cuando él busca a la madre, pero también se puede aplicar a un adulto para indicar la presencia de un sentimiento similar por estar emocionalmente cerca a otra persona. Significaticamente, el sentimiento de *amae* no se puede conseguir a través de palabras, aunque puede ser reconocido como tal en las reflexiones. También, cuando se frustra este sentimiento, puede fácilmente conducir a un desco por el mismo. Dos historias populares, una francesa y la otra americana, se cita para ilustrar la existencia de *amae*, de hecho, su importancia central, aún fuera del contexto japonés. La sicologia de tener mascotas también se puede entender en términos de *amae*. Se sostiene, por tanto, que aunque el concepto viene del japonés, es universalmente aplicable y puede dar luces sobre la vida emocional como meta principal de las investigaciones sicoanalíticas.

F reud once stated, in defending his new concept of sexuality, 'We use the word "sexuality" in the same comprehensive sense as that in which the German language uses the word *lieben* (to love)' (1971). His statement is interesting as it suggests that a concept is inherent in verbal usage. It does not follow, however, that what can easily be seen in one language will necessarily be likewise in another language. For instance, you cannot say in Japanese 'give somebody one's love' or 'fall in love' or 'make love', using each time one single Japanese word that might correspond to the English word love. This perhaps makes the Freudian concept of sexuality less accessible to Japanese-speaking people, even though it may not necessarily make the concept less comprehensive. That being the case, I hope you will not be surprised to hear that there is a concept in Japanese that bridges dependence and attachment, two concepts which are conceptually separate in English. That concept is *amae* and I shall explain how it combines the two meanings.

Amae is a noun form of *amaeru*, an intransitive verb meaning 'to depend and presume upon another's love or bask in another's indulgence'. It has the same root as the word *amai*, an adjective meaning 'sweet'. Thus *amae* can suggest something sweet and desirable. Perhaps what is most significant about the word *amae* is that it definitely links with the psychology of infancy, for we say about a baby that it is *amaeru*-ing when it begins to recognize the mother and seek her, that is to say, long before it begins to speak. Please note that *amae* here refers to the feeling of attachment that is observable. Later, when a child begins to speak, he or she will eventually learn that such a feeling is called *amae*. But that does not change the situation that the feeling of *amae* is something to be conveyed nonverbally.

Interestingly, the word *amae* can be predicated not only of a child, but also an adult when he or she displays a certain behavior *vis-à-vis* another that indicates the presence of a feeling of being emotionally close, something similar to what prevails between a baby and its mother. In other words, the assumption is that there is a continuity between children and adults so far as *amae* is concerned. Thus we may use the word *amae* to describe the relationship between lovers, friends, husband and wife, teacher and student, even employer and employee. However, it is important to remember that though one may apply the word *amae* to a person to whom one is speaking or to a third person, one cannot do so for oneself when one is actually *amaeru*-ing, like saying 'I love you', unless one is in a reflective mood to acknowledge one's *amae*. *Amae* then may not be visible to the person referred to in the same way as it is to the observer, that is to say, one may not be aware of one's own *amae*. The discrepancy between an emotion and its verbal recognition is not something unusual or rare. Rather it happens often, as we all know. However, it may be most pronounced in the case of *amae* because of its originally preverbal and nonverbal nature. At any rate, this explains, perhaps at least partially, why certain languages, like English, can manage without such a vocabulary.

I think it must be clear from what has been said above that *amae* involves a certain psychological dependence, because one who wants to *amaeru* requires another person who senses one's need and can meet it. Thus *amae* is vulnerable and, being susceptible to frustration, it undergoes various transformations. This explains, in my opinion, the existence of a rich vocabulary in the Japanese language to express variations on the theme of *amae*. I might add in this regard that the word *amae* itself sometimes meant, in old literature like *The Tale of Genji*, a certain coyness other than the meaning given above. This is an indication that the elusive and delicate quality of *amae* did not escape the attention of our ancestors. I might also mention herewith a curious fact that the Japanese as a rule are very shy of showing affection in public. The parents and their children do not embrace or kiss each other when the children are grown up. Even lovers and spouses do not. I think this shyness must be somehow related to the hidden psychology of *amae*.

Next, I want to emphasize that even though *amae* requires a generous partner for its satisfaction, it is not necessarily a passive state. *Amaeru* is an intransitive verb; therefore, it presupposes a certain capacity on the part of the person who does *amaeru*, the capacity to initiate the action leading to *amae* and to enjoy it. In other words, though *amae* indicates a feeling in the state of satisfaction, it can be felt as a desire in frustrated states. The facts about *amae* mentioned above make it a very useful word in describing the emotional life of a person, which is why it can shed light on various psychoanalytic concepts, as was shown in my earlier paper (Doi, 1989). In the present paper, I shall try to make the concept of *amae* familiar to you, just as it is to Japanese people. In order to do so, let me introduce two stories, one French and the other American. While you may not have read the stories, the scenes the stories depict may be familiar to you.

The first story is Antoine de Saint-Exupéry's *The Little Prince* (1971). The little prince comes alone to the earth and feels lonely. He meets a fox in the desert and wants to befriend him. The fox advises the little prince to tame him if that is his purpose. The little prince does not understand what 'tame' means and asks what it is. The fox explains it is to establish ties. The little prince again does not understand what it is to establish ties. The fox then describes as follows:

> To me, you are still nothing more than a little boy who is just like a hundred thousand other little boys. And I have no need of you. And you, on your part, have no need of me. To you, I am nothing more than a fox like a hundred thousand other foxes. But if you tame me, then we shall need each other. To me, you will be unique in all the world. To you, I shall

be unique in all the world. . . . (p. 80).

I think this passage describes very well how taming involves attachment and dependence. The fox then explains how taming can be accomplished:

> 'You must be very patient. First you will sit down at a little distance from me – like that – in the grass. I shall look at you out of the corner of my eye, and you will say nothing. Words are the source of misunderstandings. But you will sit a little closer to me, every day. . . .' The next day the little prince came back. 'It would have been better to come back at the same hour,' said the fox. 'If, for example, you come at four o'clock in the afternoon, then at three o'clock I shall begin to be happy. I shall feel happier and happier as the hour advances. At four o'clock, I shall already be worrying and jumping about. I shall show you how happy I am! But if you come at just any time, I shall never know at what hour my heart is to be ready to greet you. . . . One must observe the proper rites.' 'What is a rite?' asked the little prince. 'Those also are actions too often neglected,' said the fox. 'They are what make one day different from other days, one hour from other hours. . . .' (p. 84)

Now from my point of view, what is most interesting about this passage is that it describes the happy feeling that accompanies taming. And this feeling, I want to say, corresponds to *amae*. Please note that it is emphasized here that this feeling is not mediated by words, just as I stated about *amae* that it is to be conveyed nonverbally. Incidentally, there is an intransitive verb in the Japanese language, *natsuku*, which means 'to get tamed'. I think the fact that such a word exists suggests that there is a spontaneous action to invite taming, just as the fox said 'tame me', on the part of the one who gets tamed. You will see that there is a clear parallel between *natsuku* and *amaeru*, both being intransitive verbs. Namely, *amae* can be defined as the good feeling of one who does *natsuku*. One might then say that what the fox is saying in the above conversation amounts to just that. But perhaps what we should marvel at is that in order to express what this plain Japanese word *amae* means, de Saint-Exupéry had to invent a modern fable.

The second story is Paul Gallico's *Jennie* (1950). It is the story of a small boy called Peter who was one day hit by a car and went into delirium. While in delirium, he believes that he was transformed into a cat, meets a very friendly she-cat called Jennie, and they begin wandering together. The bulk of the story is about their numerous adventures, but this, though entertaining in itself, does not concern us here. What interests us is that the author calls our attention to Jennie's overlapping with his mother, for when Peter awakens from the delirium he loses the image of Jennie to his great distress, but he finds his mother at the bedside who is calling to him anxiously. He realizes then that he has not lost Jennie after all, that she is alive in his mother's love. We are given to understand at the beginning of the story that though Peter longed for his mother she was always busy with her social life, leaving his care entirely to his nanny. This nanny did not like cats and because of that he was not allowed to keep them, much as he was fond of them. One day he saw a pretty kitten outdoors, ran out to hold it and that was how he got into a car accident. So it is as if he could finally secure his mother's love by the accident. Now that he basked in her affection he understood that he had been like a hapless kitten before with all its miseries and longings. I think it is clear that the emotion Peter was driven with throughout was that of *amae*.

I hope that by introducing two stories, the psychology of *amae* will be more familiar and understandable. Is it not curious that both stories had to use animals in order to bring an element of *amae* into the picture? Of course for Japanese people, *amae* is one of those mundane things and we do not need animals to illustrate it. But there is one revealing episode in this regard. Many years ago I was telling the late Professor Y. Uchimura, my former teacher, that *amae* is a unique word in the Japanese language and there seems to be none in European languages which corresponds to it. He replied at once, 'That's strange. Why, even a puppy does it.' This comment is extremely interesting. It definitely shows that Japanese people take for granted the continuity of humans and animals, let alone the continuity of children and adults, so far as *amae* is concerned. But this continuity, which is self-evident to the Japanese, is not necessarily so to non-Japanese people and that is why, one might say, these animal stories had to be written to bring home this truth. There is another important point related to why humans love to keep pets. The answer to this question seems to be obvious. I would say that they keep pets in order to enjoy vicariously the gratification of *amae*, that is to say, attachment and dependence. Now none of you will say that you do not understand why humans love to keep pets. To the extent that you do, therefore, you too have understood the psychology of *amae*.

I could perhaps stop here if the purpose of this paper were simply to relate the meaning of the word *amae*. But because this paper was written for an audience of specialists in infant psychiatry and psychology, I should at least mention that the concepts born out of recent studies, such as the mother-child symbiosis (Mahler, Pine, & Bergmann, 1975), affective core of the self (Emde, 1983), or intersubjectivity (Stern, 1985), can all be related to *amae*. Though not a recent study nor based upon the direct study of infants, Balint's (1965) concept of primary love is quite pertinent in this context. I do not mean, however, that because these concepts can be described in terms of *amae* they are superfluous. On the other hand, I also do not think that *amae* is of no use scientifically because its meaning is so broad and we now have a learned language of precise meaning. Therefore, what is the advantage of having the vernacular of *amae* for scientific discourse? Or, conversely, what is the advantage of learning new scientific concepts of infant psychology for those who are conversant with *amae*? I will say that those who are conversant with *amae* will be surprised to find the psychology of *amae* working in those areas to which the new scientific concepts of infant psychology apply. In other words, it is not quite enough to get acquainted with those learned concepts alone. One has to learn that they, too, refer to the everyday experience the word *amae* describes. Thus, by combining everyday language and scientific concepts one can enhance and deepen one's understanding and insight. One might point out here that the word *amae* is vernacular only to the Japanese and would be just as unknown to the non-Japanese as scientific language to the uninitiated. I wonder, however, if the benefit the Japanese seem to enjoy on account of *amae* cannot be shared by the non-Japanese. I think it can and that is why I have written this paper. Curiously, though it may not be curious, I confess that in trying to explain *amae* in English, I myself have learned a great deal more about it.

REFERENCES

Balint, M. (1965). *Primary love and psychoanalytic technique.* New York: Liveright.
de Saint-Exupéry, A. (1971). *The little prince.* (Translated from the French.) New York and London: Harvest/HBJ.
Doi, T. (1989). The concept of *amae* and its psychoanalytic implications. *International Review of Psychoanalysis, 16,* 349-354.
Emde, R.N. (1983). The prerepresentational self and its affective core. *Psychoanalytic Study of the Child, 38,* 165-192.
Freud, S. (1971). 'Wild' psychoanalysis. In *Complete Psychological Works, Standard Edition* (Vol.11, pp. 219-227). London: Hogarth Press.
Gallico, P. (1950). *Jennie.* London: Penguin.
Mahler, M.S., Pine, F., & Bergmann, A. (1975). *The psychological birth of the human infant: Symbiosis and individuation.* New York: Basic Books.
Stern, D. N. (1985). *The interpersonal world of the infant.* New York: Basic Books.

First published in Ethel Spector Person et al (Eds), *On Freud's 'Observations on Transference-Love',* New Haven & London, Yale University Press, 1993

㉒ *Amae* and Transference-Love

S ince this paper attempts to discuss Freud's 'Observations on Transference-Love' from the viewpoint of *amae*, I shall first have to explain what *amae* is.[1] In brief, *amae*, a Japanese word, signifying 'indulgent dependency', primarily describes what an infant feels when it seeks its mother. Interestingly, it can also be applied to an adult when that person is supposed to entertain a similar feeling of being emotionally close to another. In other words, there is a continuum between children and adults as far as *amae* is concerned. In the case of an adult one may or may not acknowledge one's *amae* on reflection, depending on circumstances.

It is important to remember in this regard that the feeling of *amae* in itself is nonverbal. It can be conveyed only nonverbally and should be acknowledged thus. Therefore it is not a manifest emotion, but rather a silent emotion. (Perhaps that is why many languages manage without a word like *amae*.) However, in frustrated states it may turn into a desire, thus entering into the formation of many emotions, such as love, envy, jealousy, resentment, or hatred. I do not want to give the impression that this is common knowledge among the Japanese, for whom *amae* is a household word. But many thoughtful Japanese find it easy to recognize the workings of *amae* in various emotions. Furthermore, it is my contention that where such a concept is lacking, one would nonetheless intuit something similar in order to make out how the mind works.

Freud begins his paper 'Observations on Transference-Love' with a reminder that the only really serious difficulties in conducting psycho-analysis lie in the management of the transference. He cites as a typical example the case of a woman who falls in love with her analyst. What should the analyst do in such a case? To reciprocate her love is out of the question, since that would mean giving up the very purpose for which the two persons came to know each other. But if the woman insists in her demand for love? To reproach her for her passion, Freud warns, would solve nothing. Should one then compromise by at least returning her fond feelings without further involvement? Freud does not approve of this either, saying that it goes against the spirit of psychoanalysis, which is founded upon truthfulness. Moreover, there is no guarantee that one can stop at fond feelings. He also calls our attention to the fact that the erotic transference becomes the medium by which the resistance to therapy manifests itself. He concludes as follows:

> It is, therefore, just as disastrous for the analysis if the patient's craving for love is gratified as if it is suppressed. The course the analyst must pursue is neither of these; it is one for which there is no model in real life. He must take care not to steer away from the transference-love, or to repulse it or to make it distasteful to the patient; but he must just as resolutely withhold any response to it. He must keep firm hold of the transference-love, but treat it as something unreal, as a situation which has to be gone through in the treatment and traced back to its unconscious origins and which must assist in bringing all that is most deeply hidden in the patient's erotic life into her consciousness and therefore under her control. (166)

Reading this passage, one would think that it contains Freud's final word on the subject. But that was not the case; he goes on at some length. For a while he seems to be taken up with proving how the patient's manifest love cannot be genuine since it serves as resistance and is also made up of repetitions of earlier reactions, including infantile ones. Then, suddenly, so it appears to me, he reverses the argument, saying that this is not the whole story. True, the resistance makes use of the patient's love, but it did not, after all, create such love. Freud asks whether there is any love worthy of that name that does not have an infantile prototype. Thus he declares that we have no right to dispute the genuineness of the transference-love, though it may be less free than love under ordinary circumstances. Having thus established the genuineness of the transference-love, Freud comes back to the fact that nonetheless it is provoked by the analytic situation. It is evident, then, that the analyst is no more justified in taking advantage of the patient in such a state than in other medical situations. Besides, it is in the nature of the illness for which the patient seeks analytic help that her vulnerability in the sphere of love is so exposed. It therefore behooves the analyst to help her overcome a crisis in her life. With this admonition Freud concludes the paper.

I hope I have not done injustice to the complexity of the subject. At any rate, I am impressed by Freud's masterly exposition whenever I read this paper. His opening statement is that 'the only really serious difficulties' in conducting psychoanalytic therapy 'lie in the management of the transference' (159). Does he then show us in the paper some safe way to deal with it? No; if anything, he confirms the difficulties. Certainly he is enlightening and even inspiring at times. I don't know if he would mind my using the word *inspiring*. Perhaps he would not, though he would object to *inspirational*, because he knows very well that what he is arguing about borders on the moral sphere, but he would not want it to be known that he is giving a lesson in morals. However, at one point, toward the end of the paper, he actually makes the following recommendation: 'For the doctor, *ethical motives unite with the technical ones* to restrain him from giving the patient his love' (169; emphasis added). Also before this sentence, in the middle of the paper, when he advocates abstinence for the patient because 'the patient's need and longing . . . may serve as forces impelling her to do work and to make changes' (165), we cannot help but read the double meaning that the message is also addressed to the psychoanalyst. In fact later he adds the following forthright statement: 'The more plainly the analyst lets it be seen that he is proof against every temptation, the more readily will he be able to extract from the situation its analytic content' (166). No doubt the point that Freud keeps belaboring is very important, and I hope that my comments from the viewpoint of *amae* will not minimize the difficulties.

There are three points I would like to discuss here. First is the phenomenology of the transference-love, 'the case in which a woman patient shows by unmistakable indications, or openly declares, that she has fallen in love, as any other mortal woman might, with the doctor who is analyzing her' (159). I wonder if Freud fully realized that such a one-sided confession of love on the part of the woman patient was more likely due to the basic rule of psychoanalysis, which stipulates that one ought to tell whatever comes to one's mind without reservation, than otherwise. True, Freud says later that the confession 'is provoked by the analytic situation' (168), but did he really mean that it was so provoked with good reason? For it is certain that the analytic situation fosters a childlike mentality. Then, will not the transference-love approximate the case of a small child saying 'I love you' over and over again to its mother? It may be of interest in this regard that Japanese children don't say 'I love you' to their mothers, not necessarily because there is no expression equivalent to this in Japanese, but rather, I believe, because they know how to communicate with each other in nonverbal *amae*. Along this line of thought one may say, therefore, that the 'I love you' of the children in Western societies does stand for *amae*. Isn't it possible, then, to assume by extrapolation that behind the transference-love of Western adults as well hides the psychology of *amae*? I believe this to be a quite plausible proposition.

This reasoning leads to my second point, the question of how to cope with the transference-love. I think Freud's view on this matter can be summed up as follows: The patient's demand for love should not be responded to, yet it deserves to be respected since one cannot dispute the genuineness of her love. Suppose that the kernel of the transference-love is *amae*, as I indicated above. Would that change Freud's injunction with regard to the management of the transference? I don't think so. I may say, however, that to understand the transference-love as an expression of *amae* would probably make it less tempting or less threatening to the analyst. What about the patient? Can that understanding be conveyed to the patient? I say it can and, as a matter of fact, should be. But the difficulty lies in the fact that this understanding cannot be given to the patient in the form of an interpretation. For if one did give an interpretation using the term *amae*, it would sound terribly condescending or even reproachful, because, as I said at the beginning of this paper, *amae* should be acknowledged only nonverbally. Still, it is possible that the patient herself will come up with the interpretation, if she happens to be a native speaker of Japanese, that it was only *amae* which drove her to behave as she did. Or she might say substantially the same thing without using the word *amae*. At any rate, in such a case the analyst cannot but agree with her, which undoubtedly will fortify her in her new insight. But what if the concept of *amae* is not known to the analyst or the patient, as in Western clinical situations? All the same, I think, something quite like an insight into *amae* on the part of the patient and its acknowledgment on the part of the analyst will take place in a successful analysis. To prove this, let me quote certain clinical vignettes from recent works by an American analyst, Dr. Evelyne Albrecht Schwaber. The paragraph quoted below is from one of her most recent papers (1990):

> A patient was talking one session without much affective colour, of different things – some memories of his mother, depriving, seductive. I was quiet; he went on. Then he said, with a sharp affective immediacy, 'I have this feeling I want you to hold me.' 'Just now?' I asked. 'Yes.' Thinking of what he'd been saying about his mother, I then asked, 'Did she ever hold you?' 'Not really,' he replied, and he spoke, poignantly, of how, when he was little, he would go into her bed and just watch her breathing while she was asleep; at times he'd put his arm around her. . . . 'What made you feel this now, to me? I wondered. 'An emptiness,' he answered, but without elaboration, and his associations went back to mother and to his girlfriend. The next session he spoke of an intense longing he'd felt the previous day, for a warm greeting from his girlfriend – a painful yearning for physical contact; he even felt it at a meeting with female co-workers, just wishing he could hug them. He talked of how terribly hurt he'd been by this girlfriend's apparent rebuffs; when he came home she seemed tired and preoccupied, while he wanted a more loving response. I wondered what might have happened that intensified this sense of hurt – since the session, perhaps? He replied, 'Something bothered me here; when I said I wanted you to hold me, you shifted to my mother. I felt you were uncomfortable. It was useful talking of my mother as I did, but you shifted right to her. You've often pointed out how I do that; now you did it.' 'Oh,' I said, 'so you left the session still looking for a hug – not met.' He agreed. (235)

I think it is quite clear that this patient's transference-love, though it had a strong erotic component, was really a manifestation of *amae*. This Dr. Schwaber implicitly understood when she said at the end, 'So you left the session still looking for a hug – not met.' The concluding sentence of the paragraph – 'He agreed.' – is very significant in this respect. It means he understood that she understood what he really meant to say. And that in itself was good enough, because what he was really hoping for was not a hug itself but to be understood in the depth of his mind.

This paper also reports another case, a woman patient, who almost came to articulate her wish for *amae*. In the transference she would become angry again and again at something Dr. Schwaber said or did not say. Dr. Schwaber tried to make sense of her experience after each such incident, but to no avail, since it did not prevent her from creating angry scenes anew. One day an idea occurred to Dr. Schwaber, and I quote the passage describing it:

Then I realized there was an element I had not addressed. The patient's way of relating was to recount an experience she'd had without any hint apparent to me that she was seeking a particular response and to become furious with me afterwards when I failed to comment about the concern which she only then made explicit. I shared my observation of this sequence with her, asking her why she made her feelings clearer to me only afterwards. And she answered: 'I want you to understand me without my having to spell it out. If you really care about me, you would know; if I have to ask, it feels like begging. Even if you then understand, it is no longer the same.' (234)

Dr. Schwaber notes following this passage that after she acknowledged this patient's confession of a hitherto hidden wish, the patient made considerable progress, enacting no more angry scenes. I am sure I could cite more examples from other analysts, but I believe that these two are sufficiently illustrative, so let me proceed to my last point.

It concerns a remark by Freud in the previously quoted passage. After he states that the patient's craving for love should be neither gratified nor suppressed and that the course the analyst must pursue is altogether different, he adds: 'It is one for which there is no model in real life' (166). If by this sentence he simply meant that nobody ever attempted what he did in ways of dealing with transference-love, I have no objection. But if he literally meant that no model existed in real life that matched his recommended course, I would have to disagree. I think the reason for my disagreement must be obvious, because I am almost (but not really) equating transference-love with *amae*. The silent acknowledgment or denial of *amae* often happens in real life, not only in childrearing, but in adult life as well. In fact, I should say that *amae* is an important ingredient in any interpersonal relationship. Thus I cannot help wondering if part of the reason Freud could not conceive of any real-life model for his recommended course might have been the unavailability of the concept of *amae* or something similar to him, at least at the time of his writing the paper under discussion.

Now my final warning. Even if the argument of this paper proves to be sound, one should not jump to easy interpretation in terms of *amae*. *Amae* is not something open for everybody to see. One has to dig deeply in order to discover it anew in each case. Therefore, the difficulties in the management of the transference as Freud saw them will continue to baffle us for a long time, whether one likes it or not.

NOTES

1.   Wisdom (1987a, 1987b) has commented on the utility of *amae* for illuminating some aspects of object relations theory. For a more thorough exposition of *amae* as a universal nonsexualized drive for close dependent affiliation, see Doi, 1964, 1973, 1989, and 1992. For a recent comprehensive cross-cultural summary of developmental and psychoanalytic contributions to the theory of indulgent dependency, see Johnson, 1992.

REFERENCES

Doi, T. 1964. Psychoanalytic therapy and 'Western man': A Japanese view. *International Journal of Social Psychiatry* 1: 13-18.
——. 1973. *The anatomy of dependence*. Tokyo: Kodansha International.
——. 1989. The concept of *amae* and its psychoanalytic implications. *Int. Rev. Psychoanal.* 16:349-54.
——. 1992. On the concept of *amae*. *Infant Mental Health Journal* 13:7-11.
Johnson, F. A. 1992. *Dependency and Japanese socialization: Psychoanalytic and anthropological investigations into amae*. New York: New York University Press.
Schwaber, E. A. 1990. Interpretation and the therapeutic action of psychoanalysis. *Int. J. Psycho-anal.* 71:229-40.
Wisdom, J. O. 1987a. The concept of *amae*. *Int. Rev. Psychoanal.* 14:263-64.
——. 1987b. Book review: *The anatomy of self*. *Int. Rev. Psychoanal.* 14:278-79.

Unpublished paper presented to the IPA Congress, Amsterdam, 1993

㉓ Psychoanalysis in a Cross-cultural Context: A Japanese View

L et me begin this paper by introducing a book titled *Understanding the Japanese Mind*. The author is Dr. James Clark Moloney, an American psychoanalyst, and the book was published in 1954. The reason that I want to introduce it at the very beginning is that it highlights, as I shall explain subsequently, those issues which should be taken up to discuss psychoanalysis in a cross-cultural context.

Dr. Moloney visited Japan twice in 1945 and 1949, both during the period when Japan was occupied by the U.S. Army. Obviously he became very interested in Japanese culture. But being a psychoanalyst, his attention was soon drawn to the development of psychoanalysis in Japan. His hypothesis was that 'understanding Japanese psychoanalytic aims would. . . . throw more light on what makes the Japanese "tick" than any other approach'. For this purpose he interviewed the then active Japanese psychoanalysts through an interpreter, corresponded with them, collected evidence from informed sources such as U.S. trained Japanese psychiatrists and also had many articles in Japanese psychoanalytic journals translated into English in order to study them carefully. Thus his book, *Understanding the Japanese Mind*, came into the world as a result of his many years of intense labor.

I don't know if this book was reviewed in the psychoanalytic circle at the time of its publication and if it was, what kind of review it received. I think it is all in all a well researched and well documented book. First of all, it is a very rare book indeed and nothing of its kind was ever published to my knowledge before and since. Undoubtedly in order to understand Japanese culture, Dr. Moloney read many books on the subject then available to him. I might mention in this regard that many excellent books on Japanese culture have appeared since then and as far as the understanding of Japanese culture is concerned, Dr. Moloney's book will not compare favorably with them. One will also have to take into account the fact that he studied Japan during the Occupation years right after Japan's defeat in the Pacific War, a time when the nationalistic wartime fervor still lingered on, however faintly. In spite of all this, however, it would be grossly unfair to him if I said that he looked down on Japan with the spirit of the Far East War Crimes Tribunal. He was not just condescending toward the

175

Japanese. He was fair enough to notice even some deplorable trends in the U.S. that 'American individualism. . . . has largely degenerated into an American myth', since young people want 'material security, first and foremost'. He also seems to have appreciated some good aspects of Japanese child rearing. Yet I have to confess that I feel a bit uncomfortable when he mentions 'the culturally enforced degradation of the Japanese individual'. I don't deny that there are some features in Japanese culture that stand for such a description. But 'degradation' is too strong a word. It is a totally negative value judgement. The very same thing may be valued positively by the Japanese depending upon the occasion. I don't want to discuss the matter further, because this paper is not meant to discuss Japanese culture per se. I mention this only because Dr. Moloney placed the above-mentioned value judgement side by side with the goals of Japanese psychoanalysis, stating that the Japanese analysts would necessarily have to go along with subjugation of individuality to societal norms and that they in fact did so.

I want to set it right once again that I am not citing Dr. Moloney's views on Japanese psychoanalysis only in order to rebut them. He may be entirely right. Reviewing the articles that appeared in Japanese psychoanalytic journals, he states that they impress him as 'superficial, naive, imitative'. That surely might have been the case. Again, to express the characteristics of Japanese psychoanalysis in one word, he uses the word 'syncretization' meaning that the Japanese psychoanalysts mix psychoanalysis and their cultural heritage without much thought. In fact he thereby might have hit the right target and the most sensitive spot. It is surely possible that his criticism applies as a whole to Japanese psychoanalysis as it was taught and practiced from the time of its introduction to Japan early in this century up to the time of his research. But then whether or not it still applies to present-day Japanese psychoanalysis is another matter and I am not going to wrestle with that question now. My purpose of introducing Dr. Moloney's book here was, as I said above, to highlight the issues that should be taken up to discuss psychoanalysis in terms of culture. Because, in my opinion, it poses a fundamental question regarding whether or not psychoanalysis is culture-bound. The question is inseparably tied up with the values which Western culture came to espouse in recent centuries, such as individualism and liberalism, or if it transcends them, in other words, is culture-free. Now if psychoanalysis is simply a science in the ordinary sense of the word like physics or chemistry, as Freud wanted to claim it was, it is culture-free and can be applied to any culture. Then you cannot quarrel with the Japanese psychoanalysts' 'syncretization'. The Japanese should be perfectly entitled to use psychoanalysis in whatever way it pleases them just as they freely use scientific technology to their great advantage. Then also, the question of 'psychoanalysis in a cross-cultural context' would be meaningless just as 'physics in a cross-cultural context' is meaningless. But the fact that our program committee set up the special discussion group on psychoanalysis in a cross-cultural context implies a tacit recognition of a certain inherent relationship between psychoanalysis and culture. Then what is it? I shall try to give my answer to this question. But before I do so I have to inform you first, however briefly, how those of us who came on the scene in the 1950s approached psychoanalysis. Because therein lies the key that eventually led me to solve the question I have just formulated above.

Perhaps the best way to explain the attitude of our generation towards psychoanalysis would be to describe my own initial reaction to Dr. Moloney's book. When I first read it in the year of its publication, I was deeply shocked. I felt that it was saying that the psychoanalysis I was then learning was so contaminated by elements of Japanese culture to the extent of losing the true spirit of psychoanalysis. The impression it left on me, therefore, was anything but the cool, judicious review of the book I tried to present above. Thus began my journey to capture 'pure' psychoanalysis as it is taught and practiced in Western countries, even transcending Japanese culture, if that is what was required. Now this is stating my personal case. But I believe many people of my generation, several of whom have been quite active since in Japanese psychoanalytic circles, approached psycho-analysis in a similar, if not exactly the same, spirit. I can see retrospectively that this was also in accord with the *Zeitgeist* that prevailed in postwar Japan, that is, the ever accelerated drive for Westernization. Now you might have found the phrase I just used, 'to capture psychoanalysis', a bit alarming. Psychoanalysis is not something you can capture, rather it is supposed to catch you. Yes, I later learned that lesson at a great cost. Also, the phrase 'transcending Japanese culture' might be questionable. Even if one would transcend one's culture, one could never escape it. I learned that lesson too. Japanese culture was not something external that I could shed, but something internal I had to grapple with. In fact it was through this arduous route that I came to a better understanding of myself, hence, curious as it may sound, though perhaps not curious at all, of psychoanalysis itself.

I think I have now given the answer to the question I raised on the relationship between psychoanalysis and culture. That is to say that psychoanalysis presupposes a critique of one's own culture. As a matter of fact, it is precisely because it presupposes a critique of one's own culture that it can claim a universal validity, in other words, it becomes a science. In this connection I would like to say a few words on the concept of *amae* which I presented in a paper at the 1987 International Congress of Psychoanalysis. Since the paper was later published in *The International Review of Psycho-Analysis*, I don't want to repeat what was said there. I only want to stress the fact that the word *amae* which is part of everyday Japanese language could grow into a universal concept only because it was founded upon a critique of Japanese culture. That is why I thought it was presentable to the international community of psychoanalysis. As a matter of fact there are a lot of parallels between the *amae* theory and object relations theory or self psychology. And if I may emphasize the strength of the *amae* theory, that lies in that it suggests the affective quality of emotionally dependent relationships and its vicissitude, thereby enriching current psychoanalytic concepts in use.

To continue the discussion on the relationship between psychoanalysis and culture, and also to reinforce the interpretation I gave on that matter, let me take up the case of Freud. I stated before that Dr. Moloney's book could suggest that psychoanalysis as it is taught and practiced in Western countries is inseparably bound to cultural values such as individualism and liberalism. It is true that Freud was able to create psychoanalysis only in secular modern Europe. Thus perhaps psychoanalysts would also prosper most in a similar ambience. But this does not mean that Freud was just a champion of the modern bourgeois society. Rather he even aimed at a radical, almost subversive critique of the bourgeois cultural mores. One can say that his sexual theory was born precisely because of this critique. His almost defiant avowal of atheism also can be properly understood only from that angle. In other words, because Freud rested his creation of psychoanalysis squarely upon his critique of modern Western culture, it could claim a certain universal validity, thus reaching beyond Europe even to us Asiatics. I want to remind you here of Lionel Trilling's famous lecture, 'Freud and the Crisis of Our Culture' given in 1955 to commemorate the Freud Anniversary. In this lecture Trilling rightly pinpointed Freud's acute awareness of tension inherent in our modern culture.

I think I have made it quite clear that psychoanalysis presupposes a critique of one's own culture and it is in this spirit that one can talk about 'psychoanalysis in a cross-cultural context'. In order to avoid misunderstanding, however, let me say parenthetically that a critique of one's own culture does not mean its full, all-round understanding. A critique is by definition one-sided. It singles out for critical analysis a hitherto neglected aspect of one's culture that promises to be relevant to the issue under consideration. That is why a critique of one's own culture can claim validity beyond cultural boundaries. With this caveat I shall now turn to one more very important problem which confronts us psychoanalysts when attempting to examine the interface between psychoanalysis and culture. That is, psychoanalysis is no longer just one discipline among others. It is now a large establishment, international in scope. And if it is an establishment, it has a culture of its own. Then what can we make of it? I am of course thinking of the International Psychoanalytic Association. One can say that it ranks as one of many professional associations. But does another exist quite similar in kind to it? I think there is none. It is *sui generis*. When I was thinking of this question, I recalled one very interesting remark Freud made in one of his letters to Oskar Pfister, his Christian friend. It runs as follows: 'I do not know if you have detected the secret link between *the Lay Analysis* and *the (Future of an) Illusion*. In the former I wished to protect the analysis from the doctors and in the latter from the priests.' Now my proposition is that one can read this remark of Freud's as an admission that psychoanalysis borders on medicine as well as on religion and the boundaries can be murky. I think the boundary between psychoanalysis and medicine, including psychiatry, may not be as problematic, though it can be, and I shall not discuss it here. But the boundary between psychoanalysis and religion is very problematic and it has a bearing on the very culture that prevails in our Association. I shall take that up for discussion.

Now for the purpose of our discussion 'The Future of an Illusion' is not suitable, because Freud draws such a sharp line between psychoanalysis and religion as to foreclose further discussion. I think his earlier paper, 'The Future Prospects of Psychoanalytic Therapy' is more appropriate, since the not quite clear boundary between psychoanalysis and religion is more noticeable there. After mentioning his hopes for further developments in psychoanalytic technique he states as follows:

> I have said that we had much to expect from the increase in authority which must accrue to us as time goes on. I need not say much to you about the importance of authority. Only very few civilized people are capable of existing without reliance on others or are even capable of coming to an independent opinion. You cannot exaggerate the intensity of people's lack of resolution and craving for authority. The extraordinary increase in neuroses since the power of religions has waned may give you a measure of it.

It is apparent that here Freud juxtaposes authority and dependency need.

Also, he seems to suggest that psychoanalysis steps in where religions leave off. He of course takes great care not to give an impression that psychoanalysis functions as a substitute religion. Psychoanalysis has to do with intellect, not with emotions like religions, as Freud again made it amply clear by his almost lyrical dictum in 'The Future of an Illusion':

> The voice of the intellect is a soft one, but it does not rest till it has gained a hearing. Finally, after a countless succession of rebuffs, it succeeds.

Yet, in spite of all this optimism for the sake of the intellect, it was evidently inevitable that psychoanalysis would become deeply involved with the issues of authority and dependence. That is not only in the therapeutic relationship, but in the organization of the Psychoanalytic Association as well. One telling evidence can be found in Freud's polemical essay, 'On the History of the Psychoanalytic Movement'. Discussing why Adler and Jung had to leave the Movement and asking himself if their dissension could be accounted for analytically, he makes the following significant statement: 'Analysis. . . . presupposes the consent of the person who is being analyzed and a situation in which there is a superior and subordinate.' What he wants to say is that because of this presupposition analysis is not suitable for polemics. Then he exerts his very authority in determining what is psychoanalysis and what is not. After all, in his words, 'psychoanalysis is my creation'. Thus he entrusted those who were faithful to him with the task to propagate his creation. In other words, the Psychoanalytic Association became the guardian of Freud's legacy and in fact still is. That is why, in my view, the Psychoanalytic Association is different from all other professional and scientific associations. It resembles religions in this very respect even though it may rightly emphasize its irreligious stance.

I think many facets of our Association, which often become stumbling blocks to those who don't belong to it or sometimes even to those who do belong, become comprehensible from the viewpoint I presented above. For instance, its strict requirements for membership, its hierarchical structure, the sharp distinction between those who belong and those who don't, hence, the accentuated sense of belonging. While I was thinking of these features of our Association which distinguish it from others, I was suddenly struck by a striking resemblance between this institutional form of psychoanalysis and the traditional pattern of various Japanese organizations. I mean the *iemoto* system in Japan, which usually refers to the organizational pattern of schools of traditional arts such as Japanese music, dance, flower arrangement, Noh, tea ceremony, etc. They faithfully carry on the tradition of their respective founders with a large number of followers under the tutelage of accredited teachers. Professor Francis L. K. Hsu, an American anthropologist of Chinese origin, wrote a book, *Iemoto: the Heart of Japan* in which he argues that this *iemoto* principle, a kind of pseudo-kinship, permeates through the entire Japanese society, not only those called by that name. He reached this conclusion by comparative studies of Japan, the U.S., China and Hindu India. He indicated that if Japan is characterized by *iemoto*, the U.S. is by clubs, China by clans and Hindu India by castes. I think his argument is quite convincing.

What I have just affirmed will contradict what I stated above that the Psychoanalytic Association differs from all other professional and scientific associations. But when I made that statement I was thinking only of those associations originally developed in Western countries. It didn't occur to me then to compare the institutional form of psychoanalysis to Japanese models. Thus starting from Dr. Moloney's critique of Japanese psychoanalysis I have now come full circle. I wonder what he would think, were he still alive, of my unexpected conclusion that the Psychoanalytic Association is akin in spirit to the traditional Japanese organization. This conclusion, if it is right, does suggest that we are only human in spite of different cultures we are born into, that we have, after all, more in common than meets our eyes. With this final comment I shall close my presentation.

REFERENCES:

Doi, T. (1989). The concept of *amae* and its psychoanalytic implication. *Int. Rev Psycho-Anal.*, 16:349-354.
Doi, T. (1993). *Amae* and transference-love. *On Freud's 'Observations on Transference-Love'*, edited by Ethel Spector Person, Aiban Hagelin & Peter Fonagy, Yale University Press,

pp.165-171.

Freud, S. (1910). The future prospects of psychoanalytic therapy. *S.E.* 11, p. 146.

Freud, S. (1914). On the history of the psychoanalytic movement. *S.E.* 14, p.49 & p.7.

Freud, S. (1927). The future of an illusion. *S.E.* 21, p.53.

Freud, S. (1928). *Psychoanalysis and Faith – Dialogues with the Reverend Oskar Pfister*, New York, Basic Books, Inc., 1963, p. 126.

Hsu, F. L. K. (1963). *Clan, Caste and Club*, Princeton, D.Van Nostrand Co., Inc.

Hsu, F. L. K. (1975). *Iemoto: the Heart of Japan*, Cambridge, Schenkman Pub. Co.

Moloney, J. C. (1953). Understanding the paradox of Japanese psychoanalysis. *Int. J. Psycho-Anal.*, 34:291-303.

Moloney, J. C. (1954). *Understanding the Japanese Mind*, New York, Philosophical Library.

Trilling, L. (1955). *Freud and the Crisis of Our Culture*, Boston, The Beacon Press.

Foreword first published in David W. Shwalb, Barbara J. Shwalb (Eds), *Japanese Childrearing: Two Generations of Scholarship*, New York & London, The Guildford Press, 1996

㉔ Foreword to *Japanese Childrearing*

I t is a great honor and pleasure to be asked to write a foreword to *Japanese Childrearing*. I think the editors asked me to do so because I am acquainted with all the contributors. As a matter of fact, I have met all the authors of the seven leading chapters. We belong to the same generation, having become professionally active in the early 1950s. Although I never engaged in rigorous research myself, being an M.D. and primarily a clinician, our paths often crossed in the past precisely because of my cross-cultural interest, aroused by my study in the United States in the 1950s.

I think a few words are called for to explain my close relationship to William Caudill, whose pioneering studies of Japanese childrearing are well summarized by Carmi Schooler in the present volume. I had the good fortune to be introduced to Caudill when he first visited Japan in 1954, and at once became his consultant and colleague. This relationship continued until his untimely death in 1971. We used to discuss many things about Japanese culture, and he showed great interest in, among other things, my developing ideas on *amae*, which I interpreted as something that characterizes interpersonal relationships in Japan. Since the word may not be familiar to many readers, let me explain it briefly. It signifies indulgent dependency, primarily indicating what an infant feels when it seeks its mother, though *amae* can be applied to an adult who is supposed to entertain a similar feeling of being emotionally close to another. Understood in this way, the psychology of *amae* is not confined to the Japanese, yet the word is Japanese and the existence of such a word and its related rich vocabulary may well be indicative of Japanese culture.

In my opinion it was Caudill's interest in *amae* and its possible roots in childhood that induced him in his later years to study Japanese childrearing closely. It was he who offered me the first opportunity to present my ideas on *amae* in English, by inviting me to speak at a symposium on culture and personality that he organized and chaired at the Tenth Pacific Congress in 1961. The paper I read then, '*Amae*: A Key Concept for Understanding Japanese Personality Structure', later became widely known among those interested in Japanese studies. I might add that it was also Caudill who introduced the Vogels to me when they first came to Japan in 1958, thus contributing to the enduring, fruitful relationship that has since developed between us.

I hope it will not be considered improper to begin this foreword by emphasizing my personal relations with some of the authors; rather, it may be very significant. I do so because it seems to me that all the chapters in this volume, though they differ in methodology and object of study, converge on one point: the overwhelming importance of personal relations in Japan. One may say that what they each study and describe are, after all, the different aspects of personal relations in Japan. For instance, Carmi Schooler points out, citing the work of Caudill and others, that Japanese childrearing tends to strengthen the mother-infant bond, which undoubtedly sets the pattern for subsequent personal relations. George A. DeVos calls attention to the cultivation of social sensitivity that characterizes Japanese behavior on various levels. Betty Lanham found it remarkable that Japanese parents insist on always making the children understand the 'whys' in disciplining them. And Suzanne Vogel's chapter is especially interesting in stating that the understanding of *amae* was instrumental in orienting her in the process of mingling with the Japanese families, who became the object of her conjoint study with Ezra Vogel.

I think the preceding examples clarify what I meant by the statement that all the chapters included here evaluate and describe personal relations in Japan in one way or another. But I wonder if this inclusive viewpoint is acceptable to all the contributors. Some might argue about the advisability of comprehending all the different studies by one and the same concept; I would maintain that it is advisable to do so because one can then compare and even integrate them. All the same, it is also possible to contend that personal relations should be no less important in Western societies. I agree, but I maintain that there is a certain quality to Japanese personal relations, and that quality corresponds to what I named *amae*. To avoid misunderstanding, let me repeat what I said above: The psychology of *amae* is not confined to the Japanese. It can be understood by the non-Japanese, though it would be expressed differently in English, depending upon the situation to which it refers. But *amae* as something ubiquitous in personal relations is peculiarly Japanese, and it may he defined as the implicit common expectation of apparent readiness between people to please and serve each other.

Again, I am not saying that such expectations may never be encountered in Western societies. They are encountered, but only on rare occasions, and perhaps only in special personal relations for that matter. I think this fact must be related to the lack of a word like *amae* in European languages. There is no need for such a word, and thus no corresponding concept, no social recognition. In other words, one might just as well have said that *amae* simply does not exist there. That is what I felt keenly when I first lived in the United States. So one can say that I discovered the importance of *amae* only by living abroad, that is to say, only when and where it was missing. The concept of *amae* thus became the cornerstone of my psychiatric and psychoanalytic studies. Incidentally, this fact of appreciating one's own culture while living in another culture is very interesting, and should underlie all cross-cultural studies. One may even state that in studying a different culture one really studies one's own culture *in absentia*. I would naturally like to ask the American contributors to this volume what they learned about their own culture by studying Japanese culture.

Needless to say, I have enjoyed reading all the chapters presented here and have been very stimulated by them. I sincerely hope that the excitement I have had will be shared by all the readers of the present volume. I assure you that it will be useful not only to non-Japanese people who are curious to know what makes the Japanese tick, but also to the Japanese who want to have a more objective perspective about themselves or simply to know how they have been observed. Finally, I hope that knowing about the Japanese will also encourage readers to reflect upon the culture into which they were born and with which they have lived to this day.

Unpublished paper presented at the Panel on 'Amae, East and West', the IPA Congress, Santiago de Chile, 1999

㉕ *Amae* and the Western Concept of Love

I t is true that the reason for my initial interest in *amae* lay in the fact that its unique concept seems to indicate the characteristics of interpersonal relationships in Japan. But it has also been my belief from the beginning that the psychology of *amae* may claim universal interest nonetheless. That is why I presented my first English paper titled 'Japanese Language as An Expression of Japanese Psychology', in which I explained the meaning of *amae* among others, on the occasion of the First Western Divisional Meeting of the American Psychiatric Association in 1955. It was my good fortune indeed that Frieda Fromm-Reichmann was then in the audience. She expressed interest in what I had to say, inviting me later to give a talk on the same subject to a small group gathered at the Center for Advanced Studies in Behavioral Sciences in Palo Alto where she was in residence at that time. She was indeed the first non-Japanese psychiatrist who came to notice the significance of *amae*.

I think it is known to those who followed my work on *amae* in English that I subsequently related it to various psychoanalytic concepts in my writings, notably in that paper I presented at the 35th International Psychoanalytic Congress in Montreal, 1987, titled 'The Concept of *Amae* and Its Psychoanalytic Implications'. I shall not repeat here what I wrote there. I rather want to focus in this paper on the psychology of *amae* operating even where the concept of *amae* is not known. In other words, I want to show that *amae* may be detected in those cases where one would suppose the operation of love, but not of *amae*. This seems to be contrary to what I did in the paper I mentioned above, because there I deliberately tried to bring out the distinctive features of *amae* against what is usually meant by love. In this paper I shall instead call attention to the fact that love and *amae* may overlap more often than not.

One more caution. Since I am presenting this paper to the audience that does not have the concept of *amae* in their native languages, I naturally want to emphasize that the psychology of *amae* may exist even without being recognized as such. But in saying this I do not mean that in Japan where everybody is supposed to know what *amae* is, anybody can and does own up to one's *amae* when one is in such a state. That is not the case at all. Remember that *amae* by definition is something that takes place non-verbally. In fact only the observer can call it as *amae*. This is most typically

185

exemplified by a small child when it seeks its mother, but the same situation will prevail with adults when they take someone for granted or rely on someone's favor as warranted. They themselves seldom realize that they are engaging in *amae*. Hence it is only natural that *amae* is susceptible to repression or denial. Incidentally that perhaps explains why many languages can get by without such an explicit vocabulary.

Let me first cite an example from the non-analytical literature to show that *amae* is indeed implied at times when you might think that you are talking about things related to love. The author I want to quote is C. S. Lewis who wrote *The Four Loves*, an excellent treatise on love. He begins the Introduction with a distinction between Gift-love and Need-love and states as follows:

> First of all, we do violence to most languages, including our own if we do not call Need-love 'love'. Of course language is not an infallible guide, but it contains, with all its defects, a good deal of stored insight and experience. . . Secondly, we must be cautious about calling Need-love 'mere selfishness'. *Mere* is always a dangerous word. No doubt Need-love, like all our impulses, can be selfishly indulged. A tyrannous and gluttonous demand for affection can be a horrible thing. But in ordinary life no one calls a child selfish because it turns for comfort to its mother; nor an adult who turns to his fellow 'for company'. Those, whether children or adults, who do so least are not usually the most selfless. Where Need-love is felt there may be reasons for denying or totally mortifying it; but not to feel it is in general the mark of the cold egoist.

I think it must be clear from the above quotation that what C. S. Lewis calls need-love corresponds to *amae*. In this regard one may think of the usage of 'lovable' as well. It certainly does not refer to the one who is able to love, rather to a person who is worthy of being loved, hence the one who is susceptible to *amae*. So if Lewis is right in calling our attention to the importance of need-love as a necessary ingredient in the concept of love, then we have to conclude that anyone who discusses love will also bring the question of need-love or *amae* into his discussion. This certainly seems to apply to the case of Freud.

Freud postulated, in his attempt to analyze forms of abnormal love, 'two currents whose union is necessary to ensure a completely normal attitude in love'. They are the affectionate and the sensual current and he stated about the former as follows:

> It springs from the earliest years of childhood; it is formed on the basis of the interests of the self-preservative instinct and is directed to the members of the family and those who look after the child.

I think it is clear from his description that what Freud meant by the affectionate current corresponds to what Lewis called need-love, hence, *amae*. But Freud did not make much of this component of love in his later writings because he came to subsume it under the newly formulated concept of narcissism. So much so that it became customary among psychoanalysts to refer to the desire to be loved as narcissistic. Freud stated as follows:

> The primary narcissism of children which we have assumed and which forms one of the postulates of our theories of the libido, is less easy to grasp by direct observation than to confirm by inference from elsewhere. If we look at the attitude of affectionate parents toward their children, we have to recognize that it is a revival and reproduction of their own narcissism, which they have long since abandoned.

There is another statement of his to the same effect:

> This situation is that of loving oneself, which we regard as the characteristic feature of narcissism. Then, according as the object or the subject is replaced by an extraneous one, what results is the active aim of loving or the passive one of being loved, the latter remaining near to narcissism.

This is not a place to review Freud's concept of narcissism. But it may be safe to say that it represented for him an ideal state which exists at the beginning of life and to which one aspires throughout one's life. Then both the attitude of affectionate parents toward their children and the need of children to be bestowed such affection would be only a function of original narcissism. No doubt Freud had reasons for reasoning in these terms. It seems to me, however, that this reduces an essentially interpersonal process to one person psychology. It would certainly diminish the importance of need-love, if not love itself. For practical purposes, one may also say, it has an advantage of mitigating the vulnerability in loving, since it implies that what is important is to love and not to be loved. Interestingly, this mind-set agrees with the modern trend of exalting liberty and independence by all means possible, the *Zeitgeist* that Freud surely shared.

In this connection I would like to quote here Erich Fromm's celebrated essay, *The Art of Loving*. He states at the very beginning of the essay as follows:

> Most people see the problem of love primarily as that of being loved, rather than that of loving, of one's capacity to love. Hence the problem to them is how to be loved, how to be lovable.

It is interesting to note that he rests his argument upon the same fact as C. S. Lewis did that people usually don't distinguish between gift-love and need-love. But he, unlike Lewis, treats the latter negatively. Thus he talks about the capacity to love, but not a capacity for, being loved. In other words, his position exemplifies the modern trend of elevating gift-love while downgrading need-love. It must have been against such background that C. S. Lewis felt it necessary to clarify the importance of need-love. Furthermore, this way of downgrading need-love, in my view, most likely goes far back in Western thought. For instance, one may identify its early sign even in Aristotle. One sentence in his *Nichomachean Ethics* reads as follows: 'Most people seem, owing to ambition, to wish to be loved rather than to love, which is why most people love flattery.' I contend, furthermore, that this tendency of downgrading need-love was reinforced, if anything, by the influence of Christianity in the Western culture.

It is perhaps no wonder under these circumstances that it was only Michael Balint among the early psychoanalysts who recognized need-love as an independent factor to be reckoned with in mental life. As a matter of fact this became central to his thinking since he proposed that the primordial object-relation consists in needing to be loved, first and foremost. The Freudian concept of narcissism as an ideal prototype had to be discarded. It then became just a descriptive term denoting a secondary state. He first called need-love 'passive object love' in accordance with Ferenczi. But later he preferred to call it 'primary or primitive love', lest passive object love should imply pure passivity. Now this notion of his seems to me to be truly identical with the concept of *amae* as I indicated in my Montreal paper. His reasoning makes perfect sense as far as I am concerned. But I regret that it is not widely accepted among contemporary psychoanalysts. Is that because the legacy of Freudian concepts should not be easily abandoned? Or is it because Balint's emphasis on the need to be loved is too contrary to the prevailing ideology of the modern world that extols the virtue of gift-love at the expense of need-love?

I want to call your attention in this connection to one more curious fact. It concerns a close parallel between Heinz Kohut's self psychology and the theory of Michael Balint. As I see it, what Kohut calls self-object needs should correspond to what Balint specified as 'passive object love' or 'primary love'. But neither Kohut nor his followers seem to have noticed this correspondence. Of course this is understandable if Kohut developed his theory independently of Balint or even without ever reading him. I also do not want to deny that the emphasis on empathy as well as the terminology of idealization, mirroring and twinship which Kohut articulated are useful conceptual inventions. I do deplore the fact, however, that none of these terms are related to the psychology of love. It is quite possible that one reason for his not linking his theory with the psychology of love comes from the use of the Freudian concept of narcissism as a motivating force. No doubt he was inspired in this by Freud's dictum that 'the passive aim of being loved remaining near to narcissism'. But I wonder if the term narcissism is justified to replace need-love. Need-love presupposes a significant other, since one desires to be loved by that other. But if one is only motivated by narcissism, wouldn't one love only to be loved or to be in love, no matter whom one may happen to associate with? Then it remains narcissistic forever, does it not?

I maintain that narcissism and need-love can and should be differentiated. In fact I maintain it is very important clinically to distinguish between the two. True, people often confuse the two in their mind. In this regard it should be interesting to note that the Japanese word *amae* may apply to both cases in its everyday usage. That is why I pointed out in my Montreal paper that there are two kinds of *amae*, primitive restful *amae* and demanding narcissistic *amae*. It was regrettable indeed that Kohut could not come to the similar conclusion in differentiating genuine need-love from narcissism. But undoubtedly he could not have done so without criticizing first the solipsism that is inherent in the Freudian concept of narcissism.

At any rate, it is unfortunate to see that most psychoanalysts nowadays, whether Kohutian or not would not and could not think of love when they observe the kind of phenomena which Kohut specifically described. What can we make of all this? Surely this is related to the modern trend of extolling gift-love at the expense of need-love. This trend incidentally may be more extreme among intellectuals, including psychoanalysts, since need-love is no longer recognized as belonging to the domain of love. Furthermore, it seems to me that nowadays love itself is being too idolized or romanticized, if not sexualized, thus losing its natural, robust flavor. In other words, it is safe to say that in loving one loves love itself and not persons. This then is nothing but narcissism. It seems to me, therefore, that all this proves that gift-love dissociated from need-love only leads to its impoverishment or eventual cancellation. So let me conclude this paper with a plea for the importance of need-love once again hoping that the mundane Japanese psychology of *amae* would help restore the precarious balance in which the too one-sided Western concept of love finds itself at the present time.

REFERENCES

Aristotle. *Nichomachean Ethics*, Book 8, Chapter 8.
Balint, M. (1935). Critical Notes on the Theory of the Pregenital Organization of the Libido. *Primary Love and Psycho-Analytic Technique*: 37-58. New York, Liveright, 1965.
Doi, T. (1956). Japanese Language as An Expression of Japanese Psychology. *Western Speech*, Spring, 1956.
—— (1989). The Concept of *Amae* and Its Psychoanalytic Implications. *Int. Rev. Psychoanal.*, 16: 349-354.
—— (1992). On the Concept of *Amae*. *Infant Mental Health Journal* 13: 7-11.
Freud, S. (1912). On the Universal Tendency to Debasement in the Sphere of Love. *S. E.* 11
—— (1914). On Narcissism: An Introduction. *S. E.* 14.
—— (1915). Instincts and Their Vicissitudes. *S. E.* 14.
Fromm, E. (1956). *The Art of Loving*. New York, Bantam, 1963.
Lewis, C.S. (1960). *The Four Loves*. London, Fontana, 1963.

First published in Joan Raphael-Leff (Ed.) *CPS Psychoanalytic Publications*, University of Essex, Colchester, UK, 2002

㉖ Is 'Narcissistic' Pejorative?

I wonder if Freud knew that the term 'narcissism' he coined for the putative state where all currents of love originate would be used pejoratively. I think he must have been aware of the pejorative overtone of the term since in his scheme of things the origin is by nature primitive, undeveloped. Interestingly, he used the term narcissistic neurosis for the psychotic state. Also, he argued that the tenacity of one's ideal is narcissistic. Furthermore, Freud justified his postulate of narcissism as follows: 'The primary narcissism of children which we have assumed and which forms one of the postulates of our theories of the libido, is less easy to grasp by direct observation than to confirm by inference from elsewhere. If we look at the attitude of affectionate parents toward their children, we have to recognize that it is a revival and reproduction of their own narcissism, which they have long since abandoned.' (Freud, 1914, p.91) There is another statement of his to the same effect: 'This situation is that of loving oneself, which we regard as the characteristic feature of narcissism. Then, according as the object or the subject is replaced by an extraneous one, what results is the active aim of loving or the passive one of being loved, the latter remaining near to narcissism.' (p.133) Thus, whether to love others or to be loved by others, it can't escape being an expression of self-love. One may say indeed that Freud had no high opinion of humanity.

It was only Micliael Balint who took issue with Freud on the question of narcissism, since he was of the opinion that narcissism may ensue only as a secondary state following the break of one's initial object relation. I think this is a plausible hypothesis, but curiously, no other analyst seems to have agreed with him on this point. For instance, Heinz Kohut, whose theory deviated considerably from Freudian orthodoxy, resembling that of Balint in some important respect, still lets his edifice squarely rest upon the Freudian concept of narcissism. And I should say that precisely because narcissism is the sole motive, the word love is not even mentioned in Kohut's theory. As a matter of fact, in such cases, there should be no genuine love either. For one would love the other or love to be loved by him or her only for the sake of self-love. Surely narcissism should prevail!

I have been in agreement with Balint's position on narcissism since I discovered that *amae*, an everyday Japanese word, should correspond to what he described as passive object love or primary love. I have written about the subject extensively both in Japanese and English. I corresponded with Balint on this matter and even met him once to discuss it. But here is the rub. Don't think that *amae* always refers to a pristine state of being loved. On the contrary it is quite customary nowadays that one means self-indulgence by *amae*. To attribute *amae* to someone therefore can be pejorative more often than not. Thus the offended party may go to great lengths to deny it. It is apparent that *amae* here is equated with being narcissistic.

What does all this mean? Have Japanese people as a whole been under the influence of Freud all these years? Never! By no means! Because the usage of *amae* in the sense of self-indulgence can be traced far back in history, though it seems to have increased in the 20th century. It was after all a sign of the *Zeitgeist* which extolled independence even at the expense of indispensable dependence, leading to the emphasis of all-important self-love. In this regard one may then wonder if Freud himself also was not under the influence of the same *Zeitgeist* when he invented the concept of narcissism. Wasn't it more likely so than otherwise?

REFERENCES

Doi, T. (1989) The concept of *amae* and its psychoanalytic implications. *International Review of Psychoanalysis*, 16:349-354
Doi, T. (1992) On the concept of *amae*. *Infant Mental Health Journal*, 13/1:7-11
Freud, S. (1914) On Narcissism: an introduction, *SE* 14

Unpublished paper (in English) presented to the XII World Congress of Psychiatry. (Japanese version published in *Psychiatria et Neurolgia Japonica* (Seishin-shinkeigaku Zasshi, Vol.104, No.11, pp.1017-1023, 2002)

㉗ Are Psychological Concepts of Japanese Origin Relevant?

Let me say first that it took me quite a while before I decided on the title of my lecture. 'Are psychological concepts of Japanese origin relevant?' You may find this title a bit awkward. Relevant to what? Why do I want to discuss concepts of Japanese origin? As a matter of fact there is nothing new about what I am going to say today. It is old stuff indeed, because I want to discuss mainly Morita therapy and *amae* psychology, two subjects which you may have heard or read about somewhere and may already know that they are somehow tied up with Japanese culture. I take them up for discussion, however, not because of their interest for cross-cultural or comparative psychiatry. I want to claim rather that the principles underlying these two subjects are applicable worldwide. In other words, that they are relevant to psychiatry in general. You see it is seldom that such claim has been made by a Japanese psychiatrist. I may also add that the case under consideration runs against the current trend of evidence-based psychiatry which emphasizes hard 'scientific' data at the expense of soft human factors. So I am once again bewildered as to how I can present my case in a cogent and acceptable manner.

With these questions in mind let me proceed onto the main topics of my discussion. I shall begin with Morita therapy. This is a highly structured form of residential treatment for common neurotics. It was devised by Shoma Morita, professor of psychiatry who taught at Jikei Medical College in early 20th century. His view of neurosis and his method of treatment can be found with ample illustrative case material in his famous book, which was originally published in 1928 and is now available in English translation under the title *Morita Therapy and the True Nature of Anxiety-based Disorders* (State University of New York Press, 1998). His influence continues through the Morita school to this day and there is now an organization called the International Morita Therapy Association. That is one reason why I said above that you might have heard about it. But for those who don't know it and also for the sake of my argument let me draw a brief outline of how this therapy is conducted.

It consists of four stages, each lasting for several days or more. In the first stage the patient is left alone to rest in bed in a solitary room allowing no diversion whatsoever. In the second stage the patient is encouraged to do minor manual work around the house, though still prohibited from socializing. From this point on he is told to write about himself in a diary which the therapist reads every day and writes comments in the margin. In the third stage the patient is encouraged to engage in more practical work like cleaning, cooking or chopping wood. In the fourth stage the patient is allowed to do whatever he thinks necessary for his daily living. Obviously, in my view, the most important of the four stages is the first one of isolation and rest, because it is during this stage that the patient would experience a sudden lifting of anxiety which paves the way for eventual recovery. In fact only those who have this experience during the first stage can complete the following stages profitably. It was Morita's view that those who could thus benefit from the regimen of this therapy would be the common neurotics and those who couldn't would be the hysterics, severe compulsives or latent psychotics. One might say therefore that this treatment method also served as a means of differential diagnosis for Morita.

No doubt Morita established his method of treatment on the basis of many years of trial and error. According to Morita, its rationale was as follows. The patient is torn between two poles: one is the desire that things should be in some particular way he fancies and the other the recognition that, like it or not, reality is as it is. This conflictual situation, named by Morita as 'thought in contradiction', is said to be what perpetuates negative emotions like anxiety or fear once they were aroused by some stimulus. These emotions should have run their course and be dissipated if left alone and not interfered with. That is exactly what would happen to the patient during the first stage of therapy, so Morita observed. Being left in limbo so to speak the patient would first experience maximum mental pain only to be suddenly lifted from it in due time. Morita reiterated often that it was undergoing this experience which would be decisive, not any kind of persuasion by an understanding of the mechanism here described.

It cannot be denied that Morita therapy owes its special flavor to Japanese culture. For instance, its original arrangement or milieu of therapy that is reminiscent of the traditional Japanese household and this together with its seemingly rigid setup of four separate stages, these two may suggest the influence of Japanese culture. Apart from this the fact that Morita often used Zen aphorisms to illustrate the experience of liberation that happens during the course of treatment seems to indicate the direct influence of Zen on Morita therapy. This, however, Morita denied explicitly, saying that he only used Zen aphorisms for illustration. It is not known whether Morita himself practiced Zen. He must have been as well-read in Zen literature as he was in his own specialty of psychiatry. In fact one comes across many famous names in his book, not only psychiatrists but even some from related fields. Let me mention them by name: Emil Kraepelin, Ernst Kretschmer, Otto Binswanger, Paul Dubois, G.T.

Ziehen, J.M. Charcot, George Beard, Maria Montessori, William James, even Sigmund Freud. He was firmly convinced that his method was scientifically sound and should apply abroad just as well as in Japan. It was a pity that his claim was not acknowledged internationally in his lifetime. Let me make one comment in this connection about a possible similarity between Zen enlightenment and the experience of liberation in Morita therapy. Surely there exists a certain similarity and that is after all why Morita could use Zen sayings to illustrate the therapeutic experience. The key word here is 'illustrate'. 'Illustrate', but not 'explain'. If it comes to explanation, it is Morita therapy, I believe, which could explain Zen enlightenment rather than the other way around. Morita had a theory of mental anguish which was born out by his clinical experiences. Let me add one more reminder. It is the fact that only those who trusted Morita's integrity as a person were capable of benefiting from his therapy. Scientific theory alone is not effective in therapy. It needs the doctor-patient relationship as its agent. I'll come back to this important point towards the end of this lecture.

I shall now turn to discussion of *amae* psychology. I want here to take up *amae* especially because it sheds light on two important concepts of psychiatry, namely ambivalence and narcissism. But before I come to this, I shall first explain what *amae* is for those who have not heard of the word before. *Amae* is a noun form of *amaeru*, an everyday intransitive Japanese verb which primarily describes an infant when it comes close to its mother for comfort. Interestingly, it can also apply to an adult to indicate the presence of a similar feeling of being emotionally close to another. In other words, there is a continuity between children and adults as far as *amae* is concerned. One important feature of *amae* is that its feeling is not verbally mediated. It can be conveyed and responded to only nonverbally, though what goes on nonverbally may be apparent to the keen observer, thus permitting it to be so described. Another feature is that it may easily turn into a desire when frustrated. My attention was first drawn to the importance of *amae* because its meaning could not be conveyed in English by a single word, while there is a host of other words in the Japanese language relating to the theme of *amae*. I learned later that there were some technical terms in psychoanalysis which covered the same area as *amae*. But I won't bother you by introducing them. It will be enough to say here that the concept of *amae* somehow bridges dependence and attachment. Thus it is quite convenient to describe one's interpersonal relationships in terms of *amae*. In fact that is what I found myself doing almost inadvertently when I began to practice psychotherapy with Japanese patients. Of course I pondered over what I discovered, trying to make some sense out of my observations. For instance, in treating common neurotics, I have found that being frustrated in *amae* they yet entertain a hidden expectation of *amae* being fulfilled. It is this state of mind which, I am sure, underlies what Morita called 'thought in contradiction'. My study also extended to other forms of psychopathology, again in terms of *amae*. Thus what came to be known as *amae* theory was born.

Assuming that this explanation has to some degree succeeded in acquainting you with what *amae* is, let me proceed to a discussion of how *amae* is related to ambivalence. I think you will agree with me when I say that ambivalence is one of the most important concepts in modern psychiatry. I am especially impressed by the fact that from his earliest formulation of the concept Eugen Bleuler was convinced about its universal nature, even though it takes more extreme form in the case of the mentally ill, notably schizophrenics. It is as if his vision were sort of sharpened by observing schizophrenics so that Bleuler could now see what he missed before in ordinary people. One should wonder, then, if there is a common denominator for all the varieties of ambivalence. There is one indeed, and that is an element relating to *amae*. If you sort out cases of ambivalence, you will find that they invariably consist of a sentiment deriving from *amae* coupled with some negative feeling like envy or resentment. This way of looking at ambivalence has one definite advantage. It makes ambivalence more intelligible, even suggesting how it came about in the first place. It is also interesting to note in this regard that the word ambivalence is no longer just a technical term, since it came to be used widely among educated people, as if they understood its meaning instinctively without further ado. This may suggest that after all the meaning of *amae* is not too far beyond their ken in spite of the fact that the word itself is Japanese.

Next I shall take up the role of *amae* in narcissism. I am not dealing here with narcissism as the psychoanalytic concept elaborated by Freud, but simply as a common concept as is used in psychiatric nomenclature, in terms like narcissistic personality disorder. By narcissism, it seems to me, one usually means extreme self-centeredness whose vulnerability can be said to lie in the constant need to be buttressed up by others' attention or admiration. The narcissistic person therefore depends upon others for the purpose of keeping self-esteem, but most significantly he or she cannot acknowledge such dependence, detesting even the mention of dependence. So you may call narcissism twisted dependency or corrupt dependency. In terms of *amae* it is *amae* turned upon itself, because if *amae* be viable it has to rest upon a complementary relationship. It will strike you as odd then if I tell you that the word *amae* alone may sometime refer to a state of narcissism. In fact, as far as my observations go, this is often the case nowadays. I believe this usage of the word *amae* began only because Japan too has in recent years come under the heavy influence of '*the culture of narcissism*' which the historian Christopher Lasch brilliantly described in his 1979 book with that title. According to him, such narcissism is what characterizes contemporary American society. It may be quite ironical that the psychology of *amae* which Americans would have found quite alien in previous times came to haunt them in the present age from the backdoor so to speak.

I have now completed a brief outline of Morita therapy as well as *amae* psychology. I would be pleased if it struck a chord with you. Of course I should be sorry if it only gave an impression that I just presented some cultural and psychological stuff peculiar to Japanese psychiatry. I know that in today's climate of evidence-based psychiatry such things as I have called your attention to tend to be relegated to the backyard, if not neglected completely. I also notice a trend lately that shuns the age-old distinction between mental and physical illness for the sake of the much-awaited integration of neuropsychiatry. But it is a fact nonetheless that we have to deal with physical and psychological phenomena separately in examining as well as treating patients. I want to emphasize then that the cultural and psychological aspects I presented today have not been pursued for their own sake, but only because they do help to understand individual patients as whole persons. I do think therefore that they ought to interest any psychiatrist working anywhere in the world.

It is interesting to remember here that Morita himself often stressed that his method of treatment was truly scientific. In fact one might say that he himself believed in science, as every sensible person is supposed to do in this modern world. I would say that Freud was even more ambitious than Morita in this respect, since he was confident that he created a new mental science based on the pattern of natural science. In recent years this claim of his has been severely criticized and in consequence the popularity of psychoanalysis has fallen into a decline. Incidentally, we also hear that Morita therapy is not so effective as it used to be. If that is so, I wonder if that is not due to the fact that people don't trust the doctors lately as they did in times gone by, because they tend to place their faith mainly in science, more precisely in natural science. In fact the proficiency in science is so much highly regarded that the personal integrity of individual scientists or doctors no longer seems to be taken into account nowadays

This is the situation, I am afraid, that prevails in present-day Japan. I wonder if it may not be the same in the rest of the world. You see this state of affairs is hardly conducive to development of a good therapeutic relationship. Surely science alone does not teach us how to be the doctor in the doctor-patient relationship for all its advanced knowledge of brain chemistry even plus psychological sophistication that goes with it. Evidently it takes more than science to be the doctor since the doctor is bound to represent authority. Are you surprised that I introduce the word authority here? I know that people don't like it at all. But it is a fact that unless the doctor represents some authority, nobody would come to consult him in the first place. No authority, no therapeutic relationship. Of course it is not that this authority is beyond challenge. It can and should be challenged, but that again is impossible without presupposing authority. This is self-explanatory, isn't it, paradoxical as it may sound? I want to add in this connection that it was because of such nature of the therapeutic relationship that I could observe the manifestation of *amae* and its derivatives when they develop as transference phenomena.

We should perhaps pause for a moment here and question why natural science came to command such a universal respect in recent times. It is undoubtedly due to the supposed objectivity of natural science. It is taken for granted that such objectivity is the most endearing thing in our changing world. But I wonder if this claim would apply to natural science wholesale. After all, objectivity is a postulate or a matter of belief, isn't it? The objectivity of natural science can only mean that its primary goal is to be objective, namely, not to be influenced by preconception. So it happens more often than not that so-called scientific facts are, in fact, cooked up. It is thus not a contradiction to speak of objectivity in subjective matters, any more than it is to speak of subjectivity in ostensibly objective matters. In order to avoid misunderstanding, let me hasten to be more specific. By the objectivity in subjective matters I don't mean the biological substratum that underlies subjectivity. I mean thereby what should justify subjective strivings, that is to say, morality itself. I dare say it is the negligence of such morality which has muddled the subjective world of ours irreparably. As a matter of fact one would not be able to speak of personal integrity in the first place if there exist no objectively valid values to begin with. You see the word objectivity after all stands for authority according to the modern usage of the word.

I think I came a long way in discussing concepts of Japanese origin. I hope I have done justice to them as much as I could. So let me only say as the final word that it would be impossible to conduct any psychotherapy whatsoever or any therapy for that matter, whether Japanese or non-Japanese, be it Morita therapy or psychoanalysis, without ourselves being firmly grounded in the moral world. Is it perhaps banal or outdated to say such a thing in a scientific meeting like ours? What do you think? Should we not awaken to objectivity in our present mixed-up world of subjectivity? The question is not technical, not even moral in the narrow sense of the word. It is deeply philosophical. With this philosophical question I shall close my lecture.

Index of Names

General Index

Aeneid (Virgil), xi
Amae, Amaeru, ix, 9, 10, 14, 31, 32, 48, 55, 76, 80, 93, 95, 123n., 124n., 134ref., 137, 145, 147, 148ref., 150, 152, 159, 160, 161ref., 166, 169, 186, 191
  ambivalence and, 15, 48, 143, 195
  analysis of literature using the concept of, x-xii
  as a basic desire, desire to *amaeru*, desire of *amae*, 15-20, 25, 26, 48-51, 78, 79, wish to *amaeru*, wish for *amae*, 15, 16, 18, 27, 41, 48, 68, 142, 172
  concept of *amae* (*amaeru*), vii, ix-xi, 14, 16, 25, 47, 53, 64, 76, 78, 127, 140-143, 146, 147, 148ref., 163-165, 168&168ref., 172, 173, 174ref., 177, 180ref., 182, 184, 185, 188, 189ref., 191ref., 194
  feeling of, 18, 41, 68, 87, 101, 137, 142, 151, 163, 164, 169
  frustration of (in), 15, 18, 20, 48-51, 87, 93, 101, 127, 141, 194
  Japanese words closely related to *amae*, (*amaeru*), 10-12, 16, rich vocabulary regarding *amaeru*, rich vocabulary concerning *amae*, 17, 18, 33, 79, 140, 165, 182, 194
    See also *Higamu, Kodawaru, Sumanai, Suneru* and *Toraware*.
  narcissism and, 138, 142, 143, 188, 191, 195
  ninjō/giri and, 48, 49
  on and, 19, 20
  psychology of *amae* (*amaeru*), *amae* psychology, ix-xi, 14, 16, 19, 25, 33, 67, 68, 79, 87, 92, 124n., 140-144, 151, 165, 167, 171, 182, 183, 185, 189, 192, 194-196
  theory of *amae*, *amae* theory, xii, 127, 177, 178
  Uchimura Kanzō and frustrated *amae*, 101, 102, 124n.
Amae de bungaku o toku (Analysis of Literature using the concept of *amae*) (Hirakawa and Tsuruta), x
Amae no kōzō (Anatomy of Dependence) (Takeo Doi), ix
Amaeru:
  See under *Amae*

Ambiguity, 81-83, 133, 153
  tolerance of, 133
  Japanese, 81-83, 153
Ambivalence, Ambivalent feelings, 15, 48, 87, 88, 105, 123n., 142, 143, 147, 152-154, 158, 160, 194, 195
American:
  mind, 149, 150
  psychiatry:
    See under Psychiatry.
Analysis of a Phobia in a Five-Year-Old Boy (Sigmund Freud), 94, 96ref.
Anatomy of Dependence, The (Takeo Doi), vii, ix, 123n., 134ref., 148ref., 154, 174ref.
Anatomy of Self, The (Takeo Doi), vii, 138, 139n., 154, 174ref.
Apology, 15, 66-68, 87
  love and, 66-69
  See also *Sumanai*.
Art of Loving, The, (Erich Fromm), 187, 189ref.
Attachment, 29, 55, 142, 145, 147, 148ref., 163, 164, 166, 167
  dependence and, 142, 163, 164, 166, 167, 194
Authority, 27, 28, 52n., 70, 91, 93, 95, 100, 119, 139, 155-158, 160, 161, 179, 196, 197
  of (for) psychoanalyst, 155-158, 161, 179
  of religion, 156, 158, 160

Basic Fault, The (Michael Balint), 142, 148ref.
Buddhism, Buddhist, Buddhistic, xi, 6, 19, 26, 33, 35, 42, 52n., 75, 83, 124n.
  See also Zen.

Child psychiatry, 4
Childrearing, 33, 38n., 151, 173
  Japanese childrearing, 33, 176, 182, 183
Christianity, xi, 35, 52n., 97-99, 101, 103, 105-108, 112, 113, 115, 117-121, 160, 187
Chrysanthemum and the Sword, The (Ruth Benedict), 13n., 21bib., 51n.
Closing of the American Mind, The (Allan Bloom), 149